CONSERVATIVE
vs
SURGICAL MANAGEMENT
of
FOOT DISORDERS

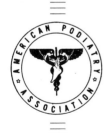

CONSERVATIVE
vs
SURGICAL MANAGEMENT
of
FOOT DISORDERS

Scientific papers presented at the
59th Annual Meeting of the
AMERICAN PODIATRY ASSOCIATION
in Denver, Colorado

Edited by
James M. Griffin, D.P.M.
Associate Editor
Louis G. Buttell

Distributed by
YEAR BOOK MEDICAL PUBLISHERS • INC.
35 EAST WACKER DRIVE, CHICAGO

Library of Congress Catalog
Card No. 73-189183

ISBN 0-87993-015-2

Distributed by
YEAR BOOK MEDICAL PUBLISHERS • INC.
35 EAST WACKER DRIVE, CHICAGO

Contents

Acknowledgment ix

Foreword xi

I. Preventive Foot Care

For the Pediatric Patient 3
  Robert W. Collett, M.D.

For the Pediatric Patient 7
  Richard P. Schuster, D.P.M.

For the Adult Patient 11
  Merton L. Root, D.P.M.

For the Adult Patient 15
  Leland G. Hawkins, M.D.

Questions and Comments 23

II. Emerging Trends in Health Care
A Challenge to Private Practice

National Health Insurance 39
  Emmett Zerr

Health Maintenance Organizations 45
  James L. Kurowski

Private Insurance Concepts in the Delivery
and Financing of Health Care 51
  James H. Hunt

Group Practice: A Challenge to Podiatry 59
  Donald C. Helms, D.P.M.

III. Practical Application of Assessment
Factors and Criteria for Surgical
Approach To Hallux Abducto Valgus

The Surgical Treatment of Hallux Abducto Valgus 63
  Stephen D. Smith, D.P.M.

Surgical Correction of Hallux Abducto Valgus 75
  Lowell S. Weil, D.P.M.

IV. Drug Interactions

Drug Interactions in the Podiatric Patient 85
  Daniel A. Hussar, Ph.D.

Drug Interactions — The Need for Careful
History Taking 97
  Samuel Moskow, D.P.M.

The Management of Reactions to Local Anesthetics 109
  S. Crawford Duhon, M.D.

V. Pre- and Post-Operative Biomechanical
Considerations In Foot Surgery

Biomechanics and Its Relationship to Foot Surgery 121
  Fritz A. Moeller, D.P.M.

Biomechanical Implications of Foot Surgery 129
  Tilden H. Sokoloff, D.P.M.

The Importance of the Physical Examination
In Podiatric Treatment 135
  James S. Miles

VI. Evaluation of Soft Tissue Injuries
of the Foot and Ankle

Panel Discussion 143
  *Milton Fulp, D.P.M., C. Robert Starks, Sr., D.O.,
  and Joseph Doller, D.P.M.*

VII. Treatment of Clubfoot — Conservative vs. Surgical

Treatment of Clubfoot—Conservative vs. Surgical 153
  Thomas E. Sgarlato, D.P.M.

VIII. Anesthesia

Local Infiltration Anesthesia 171
  Robert E. Weinstock, D.P.M.

Nitrous Oxide Analgesia in Podiatry 185
  Mark H. Feldman, D.P.M.

Intravenous Regional Anesthesia 199
  John J. McGlone, D.P.M.

IX. Mini Surgery vs. Open Surgery

Panel Discussion 207
  *Clyde Shreve, Jr., D.P.M., Earl G. Kaplan, D.P.M., and
  Joseph B. Addante, D.P.M.*

X. Four-Handed Podiatry:
Mobilization of the Podiatric Assistant

Four Handed Podiatry 221
*Charles R. Turchin, D.P.M., Ben Hara, D.P.M.,
and William Lowe, D.P.M.*

Panel Discussion 229

XI. The William J. Stickel Awards
Selected Papers

A Study to Determine the Relative Absorbability
and Wicking Effect of Certain Major Sock Materials
on Perspiration of the Human Foot 239
James A. Davis, D.P.M.

The Damaging Effects of a Disaligned Musculoskeletal System 251
Charles L. Jones, D.P.M.

Abducted and Adducted Gait Problems 271
Brian A. Rothbart, D.P.M.

Topical Control of Infection on Gangrenous Lesions
of the Extremities 291
Stanley Levine, D.P.M.

A Clinical Study of the Phalangeal Stance Reflex 295
Stanley V. Michota, D.P.M., and Franklin A. Michota, D.P.M.

Axial Rotation of the First Metatarsal as a Factor
in Hallux Valgus 305
Richard A. Maldin, D.P.M.

Author Index 321

Acknowledgment

The demand for more and better podiatric literature has grown in direct proportion to the improvements in podiatric techniques and practice and the upgrading of college curriculum and faculty.

One of the prime sources of podiatric literature is the Annual Meeting of the American Podiatry Association. In the past, a small selection of papers from the Scientific Program has been published in the Journal and, thereby, has become available to the entire membership. However, there has been a growing recognition that a compilation of the Scientific Proceedings would be a valuable addition to the average practitioner's library.

The Board of Trustees, recognizing these needs, has authorized the publication of this volume. It was compiled by electronic taping of each of the Scientific Sessions, the transcribing of these tapes, and a comparison between the tapes and the author's manuscript. The resulting consensus copy — or verbatim transcription in the case of panel discussions — was then transmitted to the author or panelist for editing or revision. It is hoped that this has ensured that each article appearing in this volume is an accurate reproduction of what was presented at the Annual Meeting.

Foreword

The changes of this decade in the field of health will be major. They may well mean that the practice of podiatry and all the other health sciences may not exist as we now know them by 1980. That these changes will include some form of National Health Insurance is no longer in doubt, but what form will this system take. What type of podiatry practice will result from it?

These will be changes which will have a profound effect on the podiatry practitioner and the profession as a whole.

In addition, the Colleges of Podiatric Medicine must continually expand during the 1970's in order to provide the manpower needed to meet the increasing demands for podiatry services.

To prepare for these challenges, changes, and firsts, podiatrists must cooperate with the other health disciplines and direct their energies towards the continued advancement of our nation's health care system.

The Scientific Program of this 59th Annual Meeting has emphasized the delivery of improved health care through a better understanding of modern technology and public need.

May this volume help all of those who are concerned with the care of patients to better meet the challenges of the 1970's.

In summary, the Association, through this volume, is attempting to make a significant contribution to podiatric literature and to the educational advancement of all those interested in podiatry and foot health.

Lawrence G. Lefler, D.P.M.

I. Preventive Foot Care

Preventive Foot Care –
For the Pediatric Patient

Robert W. Collette

This paper is directed to the prevention of foot pathology in childhood. I am sure you agree that if we can prevent some of the foot problems at this age-level there will be less difficulty when the child becomes an adult.

In considering the origins of pathologic conditions of the foot, some can be traced to the position of the fetus in utero. If the child's feet are folded under the soft tissue of the buttocks, you can get a metatarsus varus; if there is a crossing of the legs with the feet pressed against the bony parts of the leg, you can have club feet.

There are various other conditions directly related to the actual fetal position of the child; extreme hyperflexion of the foot, eversion and inversion of the foot; and, dislocation of the hip caused by the fetal position of the child as it sat in the womb before it was born, or extreme tension on the leg causing the hip joint not to be in its socket. Adduction tightness of the hips can be shown to be related to fetal positioning. Breech deliveries may contribute to pathologic hyperextension of the leg and malposition of the foot in relation to the rest of the body; twisting or torsion of the thighs may also cause pathologic conditions.

It is surprising the number of things that can be found on examination of a newborn child if one is aware of the pathologic possibilities. The child can be quite active or limp, depending often on the APGAR score when the child was born and how it has responded to the tremendous shock of coming into this world.

There are a number of reflexes we look for: the sucking reflex to see if the child has a natural movement of the mouth so that he can take nourishment; the aural reflex which is the reaction of the child to a sudden noise or shaking of the crib when he is in a prone position; the child has a grasping reflex, his hand extending and then flexing. The tonic vector reflex is very interesting. When you

Robert W. Collete, M.D., *Pediatrician, Deceased: September 25, 1971.*

turn the baby's head to one side the child assumes a fencing position with the face directed toward one side (e.g., right), the (right) hand is extended and the (right) leg is extended, the opposite limbs being flexed.

The above are some of the important reflexes normal in the newborn, and, if they persist past a certain period, may become pathological. Another reflex one sees in the newborn is a positive Babinski sign; that is, the plantar extensor reflex when the sole of the foot is stimulated. The foot of the newborn has some interesting reflexes. For example, when the heel is stroked you get plantar flexion; when the sole is stimulated you get dorsal flexion; if you stimulate the medial aspect of the foot you get abduction; and when you stimulate the lateral aspect of the foot you get adduction.

Congenital defects are, of course, of major concern in the initial examination. With special reference to the feet, the following conditions may be seen: club foot (talipes); syndactylism (webbed digits); polydactylism (extra digits); congenital absence of toes; claw foot; hammertoes which may be due to a very tight fetal position; the absence of the tibula or tibia; and phocomelia, the absence of parts or whole limbs which was seen frequently in the recent thalidomide tragedies. The named conditions are usually obvious; however, congenital dislocation of the hip may not be and it is important to diagnose the condition as soon as possible after birth.

All the foot problems we see in children are either neural, muscular, or skeletal deformities of some sort. Some may be due to brain damage which, in severe form, may be manifested as cerebral palsy or such maldevelopments as spina bifida where the nerves which go to the legs and feet may be involved. Other genetic problems may include achondroplasia (short limbs), gargoylism (Hurler's syndrome), Marfan's syndrome in which there is arachnodactyly with thin tapered fingers and toes. The only prevention of these cases is better prenatal care, genetic counseling, prevention of prematurity and brain damage at birth due to anoxia or birth trauma.

It is important, I think, to observe the limbs of a child each month in order to detect early any deformities that might show up. Therefore, one must know the various landmarks of growth and development, when a child normally grasps with his hands, when he shows inclination to roll over; before he can actually sit or crawl he has to have muscular control of turning from one side to another. The way a child sits is important in relation to his balance, the way he pulls up at 8-9 months, and the way he begins ambulation at about 10-12 months.

Walking and how a person develops his walk is so important to your profession that I feel it is important for you to know how this skill develops and to see movies of how children actually learn to walk. Their stance is wide-based to begin with and the feet are usually in a valgus position and flat footed. As they grow, the normal configuration of the foot takes place. The age at which reciprocal leg movements and tightening of the hips becomes important should be noted as the child goes through his various stages of growth and development.

Broadly considering the causes of foot problems in children, malnutrition comes to mind. There are cases of children who are malnourished though more frequently they have emotional problems or do not consume the right foods in adequate amounts. The opposite of that is obesity and you have all seen unusually obese children who, because of excessive weightbearing, have foot problems.

Other general conditions which may be associated with foot problems include rickets, which is a vitamin D deficiency uncommonly seen today, and renal rickets which is not related to vitamin D deficiency. Hypothyroidism, a hormone deficiency, can certainly be related to foot problems. Congenital heart disease in itself can cause foot problems; there may be a tremendous amount of cyanosis and a lot of pulmonary pressure. Patients with congenital heart disease may have club feet, club toes, and club fingers. Osteomyelitis, poliomyelitis, rheumatic fever, and rheumatoid arthritis are other general conditions that can cause foot problems. A condition you might not have thought about is hemophilia where hemorrhages into the joints of the knees and feet can cause considerable problems. Injuries such as burns, contractures of the muscles, and fractures can leave the foot in a deformed position if the conditions are not properly cared for at the time the injury was incurred. The earlier the diagnosis and institution of treatment for deformity the more likelihood exists that the deformity can be corrected. All the muscles and bones of the feet and legs are necessary for adequate functioning and, in addition, there must be normal hips and normal neural connections with the spine and brain.

One of the most severe conditions we see is cerebral palsy. This is due to an upper motor neuron lesion which is usually classified as (a) spastic, where the cortex of the brain is more involved; (b) athetoid, where deeper brain damage is evident in the diencephalon; and (c) atactic, which is largely due to cerebellum damage. There are variations in all of these, occurring perhaps in one individual case. Not only are motor problems involved in cerebral palsy; many cases have sensory involvement as well. Of course, there are proprioceptive and tactile senses which may be abnormal and which can affect their ambulation in addition to their abnormal motor apparatus.

Club foot is a very traumatizing condition. If diagnosed early and treated properly much unhappiness can be prevented. Flat foot is the normal condition in the newborn. Until 1½-2½ years of age the arch of the foot is not recognizable. As the child grows the muscles get stronger and the flatness disappears. Knock-knees is another condition we should be aware of and not neglect because it may cause problems with posture. Bowlegs of the non-rachitic type and also the apathic type should be recognized. Pronation is an important problem to recognize and treat early. I believe it is one of the most common causes of poor posture in children.

Limps are commonly the reason why children are brought to treatment. Often the mother believes that there are foot problems causing limping;

however, there are a number of pathologic conditions which may cause a limp. Legg-Perthes disease is one of these which may be quite disabling if not discovered and treated; this is an aseptic necrosis of the femoral epiphysis. There are various types of osteochondritis which may cause a limp in children; among these are Frieberg's disease, a disease of the second metatarsal head; Kohler's disease affecting the navicular bone; Sever's disease, epiphysitis of the os calcis; Osgood-Schlatter's disease of the tibial tuberosity; Scheuermann's disease, which is an osteochondritis of the epiphyses of the vertabrae. In a recent case of Scheuermann's disease there was only a slight limp, some back pain, and a definite difference between the length of the legs.

Recently we have become more aware of the problems of the hyper-active child, the child who has minimal cerebral dysfunction and peripheral motor problems. Generally there are a number of minor neurological abnormalities often associated with fast movements of their hands and legs. They cannot hop or skip on one leg and it is difficult for them to stand on one foot. There is a difference in their discrimination of laterality; they may be left-footed and right-handed and left-eyed, or any combination of differences in lateralities. These children almost always have some type of motor, visual, or auditory, perceptual problem. They also have a very interesting tactile sense; in fact, they are tactile defensive. You just barely touch them and they jump in overreaction. Their photoreceptive sense is impaired and they have balance problems. These children need help and should be diagnosed early. They usually do not have major pathologic foot conditions, only the general ones that children have; however, it is important for their condition to be recognized.

In my capacity as medical director of Lariman Hall, a school for retarded children in Denver, I have been impressed with the improvement that has taken place with proper treatment of these children, many of them progressing to become taxpayers and self-reliant to a certain degree. On examination of the feet of these children almost 100% have been found to have some foot pathology. It was evident that their parents, being more concerned about their behavior, forgot about their feet. In addition to a large amount of bunions, callouses and other common problems, a number of congenital abnormalities have been noted. This points up the desirability of having a podiatry consultant in the special schools that care for children with neurological handicaps.

Preventive Foot Care-
For the Pediatric Patient

Richard O. Schuster

Before considering the prevention of foot problems in children, one must consider the cause. For purposes of this discussion, we will classify causes as internal and external.

The majority of common foot problems in children are congenital in origin. In that sense, they are internal situations, and in that sense the basic problem is difficult to prevent. To oversimplify: prenatal characteristics are not always outgrown in the transition from the round nested fetus to the elongated bipedal human. As a result, the "neutral" position of the foot is not always parallel to the walking and standing surface. When body weight passes through these feet, they may sometimes break down and compensate to meet the horizontal surface. This compensation is a pathomechanical situation, and it is this part of the problem that can be prevented. In a manner of speaking, this breakdown is prevented by tilting the ground up to meet the foot by one means or another. However, the prevention of foot problems caused by internal situations is not the area I intend to discuss, I mention it only to put matters in their proper perspective. I anticipate that our colleagues will discuss the congenital aspect of preventive foot care in greater depth.

I intend to discuss some of the external situations that cause foot problems in children. This is a smaller category of foot problems, but it is nonetheless important, as it is an ever present confrontation in the office and is seldom if ever mentioned in the literature. Happily, most foot problems that are caused by environmental situations are relatively simple to prevent. Perhaps the reason that external factors have been ignored as a cause of foot problems is that they are so common that they are overlooked.

The shoe is the most important environmental factor that can cause foot problems in children (and for that matter in older groups as well). Most foot-conscious parents are more concerned about obtaining "good" shoes for

Richard P. Schuster, D.P.M., *Associate Professor of Mechanical Orthopedics, M. J. Levi College of Podiatry, New York, New York.*

their children than for themselves. Unfortunately, the "good" shoes are often the problem. Many of the so-called "good" shoes for children seem to be made without concern for the way the foot functions. (In fairness, it must be stated that the wear qualities of "good" shoes are usually excellent.) One would never think of inhibiting dorsiflexion of the ankles of a normal child — yet many "good" standard shoes are so stiff at the ball that they prevent dorsiflexion at the metatarsal phalangeal joints. Limitation of motion of any significant foot joint by a stiff soled shoe or any other device interferes with proper foot function. Tests have shown that some children's shoes may require up to 70 pounds of pressure to flex the shoe at the ball. This is often much more than the child weighs.

"Splinting" the foot of a child to a stiff, board-like sole has many effects. It may discourage or delay the walking period. Those who treat children may have been exposed to the situation where concerned parents obtained the "best" shoes after gleefully witnessing their youngster's first steps, and then were dismayed to find that the child refused to walk for the next few weeks. The fact of the matter is that the youngster is often discouraged from walking, for a while, at least, by having his feet bound to stiff leather boards. This of course is not a typical situation, but it does happen.

Much more important than a delay in the time when walking begins is the effect of stiff-soled shoes on the angle of gait. Shoes that do not flex easily at the ball act as long forward-projecting levers. It is difficult for the child to pass over these "levers" unless he "shortens" them by angling the foot to a more intoe or outtoe position. Almost invariably, a child's angle of gait becomes worse with the use of stiff soled shoes. This has been verified by measuring the angles of foot prints made while wearing stiff soled shoes, flexible soled shoes, and going barefoot.

Parents are often concerned about the appearance of intoe or outtoe. However, the importance of intoe or outtoe is its potential destructive effect on the mechanics of the foot.

Wedges on the sole of the shoe, for whatever purpose, sometimes have a worsening effect on gait angles because they act as additional sole stiffeners. We do not discourage the use of shoe wedges when indicated, but one must be aware that they could have an opposite affect. A child's shoe that is too long could have a similar effect. More than one doctor has been embarrassed by parents complaining that the child walks straighter in sneakers than in the stiff "special" shoes prescribed by the doctor. Many intoe and outtoe attitudes, and their complications, can be prevented or reduced with the use of shoes that bend easily at the ball, thereby permitting freedom of motion of the metatarsal phalangeal joints.

A word about the use of shoes on youngsters who do not yet walk. Shoes at this stage need only be protective coverings. There is really no need nor benefit in putting walking shoes on children who do not yet walk.

While we have discussed the need for shoes that flex easily at the ball, the shank of the shoe on the other hand, should be rigid. Like all other parts of the shoe, the characteristics of the shank should correspond to the function of that area of the foot. Since there is very little normal downward deflection in the midtarsal area, there should be no downward deflection of the shank beneath the midtarsal area.

The use of flexible shank shoes in children is serious. They can cause considerable damage and foot discomfort even without the presence of the usual anatomical "deformities" that one is inclined to look for. Since a flexible shank contributes little to the support of body weight, the total weight-bearing area of the foot is decreased, causing concentrations of weight in other areas. While this is a factor to be considered against the use of flexible shanks, it is not the major objection. A more important consequence of the use of flexible shanks is that it may permit the midtarsal area to "sag" or sublux through the shank causing considerably annoying symptoms of strain.

Flexible shanks are often found in imported shoes, injection moulded plastic shoes, children's house slippers, certain types of inexpensive canvas shoes, novelty shoes, and most "loafers". If for some reason, the individual insists on wearing flexible shank shoes, the situation can be improved by placing a small unnoticeable plug between the shank and the ground. Fortunately, shoe manufacturers are learning from sales experience that adults who are on their feet — waitresses, laborers, etc. — prefer shoes with rigid or filled in shanks. Unfortunately, the child's needs for rigid shanks have not become so well known to the parents or the manufacturers.

From time to time, shoes appear on the market that have rigid shanks at the time of purchase, but become completely flexible after some period of wear. In this situation, the shoe is often constructed with a wooden shank which serves only until it breaks. One can test for the presence of wooden shanks by twisting the shoe slightly through the shank area. If it makes a cracking sound, it is obviously wood.

It should be mentioned at this point that a review of records seems to indicate that the incidence of fracture of the base of the fifth metatarsal seems to be related to shoe types that have flexible shanks. The fracture often appears after a hard downward step or jump. Presumably in this activity, the ball contacts first, the heel contacts next, and the midtarsal area then "whips" through the flexible shank thereby breaking the base of the fifth metatarsal.

It could almost be a rule that once a heel is put on a shoe, the shank must be rigid.

There are other environmental influences that have an effect on the well being of the foot.

On several occasions, we have been impressed by the influence of infant walking devices on foot and leg attitudes. An infant "walker" is a cloth bucket in which the child sits. It has two holes through which the legs extend and reach the floor. This is set into a frame with four wheels so that the youngster can scoot about the room before he has learned to walk. Frequently, we have noticed that the youngsters legs are too long for the height of the seat causing the feet to function in a pronated or otherwise unnatural attitude. There is no data to verify that such a situation is harmful, although it certainly cannot be considered beneficial. In any event, a small pillow under the child will provide him with more normal use of his feet and legs.

Clothing, in certain situations, can have its effect on the development of feet and legs. Infants and youngsters up to the walking period are often put into snow suits and stretch suits in which the feet are enclosed. When these suits become outgrown and are still worn, the feet and legs are forced into a cramped and deformed attitude. No investigation has been done in this area. However, since this type of clothing is worn for hours at a time, during a critical developmental period, it seems prudent to caution parents about the possible harmful effects on the lower extremity.

A major factor in the perpetuation of some foot and leg problems is the postural habits of some children. The way one functions is influenced by one's structure. More specifically, children squat for long periods watching television or during other activities. Not all children squat and sit on the floor in the same manner. They squat the way their torsional factors permit them to squat. Since the child tends to sit on the limbs when squatting, it becomes a splinting habit affecting transverse plane "deformities" such as tibial torsion and femoral torsion. Children find it difficult to squat in any other manner than the one to which they are accustomed. When there are torsional problems of the limb in children, they should be discouraged from squatting in their usual manner. If this is not possible, they should be discouraged from squatting altogether.

Preventive Foot Care -
For the Adult Patient

Merton L. Root

Mechanical microtrauma is the major cause of symptoms and disability in the adult foot. The incidence of foot problems caused by mechanical trauma exceeds the total incidence from all other causes.

Abnormal pronation is the most frequent of the many causes of mechanical trauma. This paper will discuss the prevention of pathology which is induced by abnormal pronation of the foot during locomotion.

Pronation of the foot is a normal, necessary motion which occurs at the subtalar joint during the initiation of the stance phase of gait. Normal pronation occurs only during the initial 25% of the stance phase of gait and 4° to 6° of calcaneal eversion is all that is necessary for normal locomotion function.

Abnormal pronation is excessive pronation or pronation which occurs in the later periods of the stance phase of gait.

The normal foot must function as a rigid lever during propulsion. To become a rigid lever, the foot must be supinated at the subtalar joint. Therefore, supination of the foot during propulsion is necessary for normal function.

The abnormal foot is pronated during propulsion. It is an unstable foot. Active and reactive gravitational forces cause a shifting of forefoot bone structure during propulsion. The forefoot is not locked against the rearfoot and the foot is hypermobile and cannot function as a rigid lever.

Abnormal shifting of osseous structures during propulsion causes trauma to surrounding soft tissues. The soft tissues are fixed by the floor or by the shoe. The shifting of bone against fixed soft tissue produces abnormal shear. Shearing of bone against soft tissue during propulsion is the most frequent cause of hyperkeratotic lesions, neuromas, and bursae of the forefoot.

Hypermobility also causes osseous malalignment. Hypermobility forces joints to exceed their normal range or normal direction of motion. The result is subluxation or partial dislocation. When subluxation persists over a prolonged

Merton L. Root, D.P.M., *Professor of Podiatric Orthopedics, California College of Podiatric Medicine, San Francisco, Calif.*

11

period, functional adaptation of bone to the subluxed position will occur. Hypermobility results in joint deformities such as hammer toes, hallux abducto valgus deformity, tailors bunion, and flat feet.

In the adult, prevention of the common foot symptoms and deformities comprises two categories. These are:

1. Early detection of deformity to eliminate trauma which would eventually lead to symptoms if untreated
   and

2. Elimination of symptomatology as it first becomes evident by conservative means to prevent eventual surgery which may become necessary if the cause of trauma is not eliminated.

Much of the potential symptomatology in the adult foot can now be prevented. Furthermore, symptomatology can be alleviated by conservative care if that care is adequate and initiated early.

Preventive foot care requires two basic changes in the podiatrists' attitude before preventive foot care in the adult can become universal.

First, the practitioner must avail himself of the latest knowledge concerning the causes of abnormal pronation and how to eliminate them.

Secondly, the practitioner must reassess certain ingrained attitudes which act as a mental block to providing adequate preventive medicine. These attitudes which presently impede the progress of preventive care for the foot may be summarized as follows:

1. *Shoes are the cause of foot deformities and symptoms!* Such an assumption is scientifically unsound. Malfunction of the foot causes most traumatic symptoms. The shoe may aggravate but does not cause foot problems. A malfunctioning foot changes size and shape as it bears weight during locomotion and no shoe can fit properly. Shoe fitting and style are no problem for the individual with a foot which functions normally.

2. *Pain is the only justification for treatment of a foot problem!* Such a concept leads to loss of valuable time when correction of a malfunctioning foot is most easily accomplished. Considerable bone deformity and soft tissue trauma has occurred before pain develops. It takes much longer to reverse a deformity than to prevent one.

3. *The patient is too old to be treated except by palliation!* This concept is unfair to most elderly people. If motion is present in the major functional joints of the foot, abnormal pronation and the trauma it produces can be eliminated in most cases. Some of the most gratifying results have been accomplished in patients beyond the 5th and 6th decade of life.

4. *Most children are born with perfect feet!* Such a statement can still be seen in most literature disseminated to the public. Most children are *not* born with perfect feet or legs. The newborn is only a partially developed biped. Unless many developmental changes occur from the hip to the foot, the child would find it most difficult to ever stand and walk. Many minor and some major structural deformities are present at birth. These congenital deformities are often hereditary and preclude normal foot function throughout the life of the individual unless treatment is rendered.

How can the podiatrist provide preventive foot care for the adult? He can begin by first learning about normal structure and function of the foot. Then he can learn about the congenital and developmental abnormalities which have been identified and study their effect upon function. Next, he can develop the art and techniques necessary to adequately examine the lower extremities. Finally, he can learn to use those techniques which effectively control or prevent abnormal function of the foot.

Such knowledge is now available. Biomechanics is the newest science of medicine which is unlocking the secrets to malfunction of the foot. Biomechanics has rapidly outmoded past medical education pertaining to the foot. Even basic anatomy provides an outmoded, false impression of muscle and joint function. Unfortunately, the term biomechanics has become popular. It is fashionable to refer to biomechanics as the "in" thing.

Biomechanics is a new basic science of medicine. It does nothing more than provide an understanding of structure and function. Biomechanics won't cure anything. The doctors' knowledge and skill are necessary to cure or prevent illness or disease.

Through the study of biomechanics, the podiatrist can acquire the knowledge and skills to prevent many of the foot conditions which in the past have been accepted as chronic and incurable. Preventive foot care is best initiated in the child, but age, any age, does not preclude the improvement of foot function or the prevention of symptoms so long as adequate joint motion is present.

The public has the right to be informed and should be informed about the causes and prevention of foot disability. The podiatrist should assume the personal responsibility to recommend preventive foot care whenever he sees signs of impending pathology. It should be left to the patient to decide whether or not he will accept the doctors' recommendation. Under no circumstances should the doctor assume the patient is disinterested in prevention. All too often the doctor makes the decision for a totally uninformed patient to the patients' detriment.

Naturally, the doctor himself must be sufficiently knowledgeable to recognize impending foot pathology before he can ever fulfill his responsibility to the patient.

Preventive Foot Care
For the Adult Patient

Leland G. Hawkins

Gunshot Wounds

Gunshot wounds of the foot have become rather common civilian occurrences. The common caliber pistols, (.22, .38, .45 cal.) carried for self-protection, have an approximate low-missile velocity of 1,200 feet per second in contrast to the high-velocity missiles or shrapnel which cause military casualties. The surgical management of gunshot wounds in civilian circumstances is different than on the battlefield (Fig. 1). Debriding the skin edges of the wounds of entrance and exit is essential. Nothing need be done with the fragments that you see loose in the center of the foot. If they are subcutaneous in a weight-bearing area the fragments should be removed. The patient is placed on antibiotics and the foot is elevated. Infection rarely develops in the wound tract of low-velocity missiles or shotgun wounds. My message in this type of case is not to excise widely the soft tissues of the foot but rather debride only the skin edges, use antibiotics, elevate the foot, and treat until skin closure and fracture union.

Metatastic Carcinoma

A 50-year-old man complained of foot pain which he related to a specific injury four weeks earlier. Periosteal new bone along the shaft of the second metatarsal was found (Fig. 2). The diagnosis is a stress fracture. I applied a short-leg walking plaster and asked the patient to return for follow-up. Three weeks later he still complained of pain. I prescribed analgesics and asked him to return again in three weeks. I resisted the idea that he might have metatastic disease since I had been taught that this rarely happens distal to the knee or elbow.

However, when he returned again and after asking a few simple questions like "Do you cough?", "Do you smoke?", "Have you lost weight recently?", the

---

Leland G. Hawkins, M.D., *Chief, Division of Orthopedic Surgery, Denver General Hospital, Denver, Colorado.*

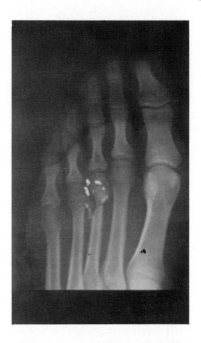

Figure 1.

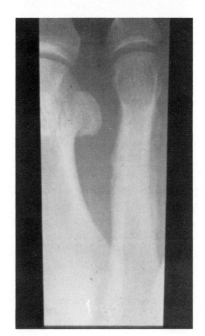

Figure 2.

pattern became obvious and a chest x-ray revealed carcinoma of the pulmonary parenchyma which required lobectomy. A biopsy at that time of the metatarsal proved the lesion to be metatastic from the lung.

Stress Fractures

A woman referred to me for excision of a Morton's neuroma presented with swelling on the dorsum of the foot.

A stress fracture of the third metatarsal was seen on x-ray (Fig. 3.). The foot was placed in a plaster cast but the pain persisted for about six weeks. She continued to have swelling on the dorsum of her foot and a localized area of tenderness over the extensor tendons to the fourth toe. The patient had been previously injected with steroids to resolve her Morton's neuroma, and additionally had a very low-grade rheumatoid arthritis which confused the clinical picture. It was decided to surgically explore this very local tender area on the dorsum of the foot in the region of the extensor tendons. During surgery another stress fracture of the fourth metatarsal was found (Fig. 4) in addition to the mass of unresorbed steroids adjacent to the extensor tendons. Later this patient had a third stress fracture of the second metatarsal. She has a rigid hindfoot and some limitation of pronation from her low-grade rheumatoid

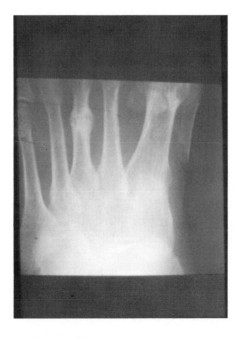

Figure 3.

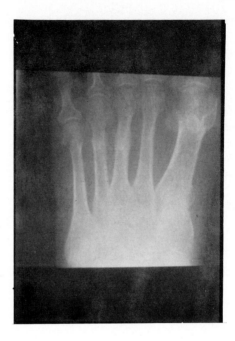

Figure 4.

arthritis. I would like to have some explanation for three stress fractures in one patient.

Superficial Ulceration of the Foot

Today a number of preparations are commonly used in the treatment of superficial ulcerations of the feet; for example, local steroids, proteolytic enzymes, local antibiotics, and antiseptic solutions such as benzalconium chloride, hexachlorophine. Iodiphore preparations are organic iodides which release about 1% free iodine. This preparation admirably serves the purpose of sterilizing the skin preoperatively in most operative procedures done today. To sterilize the ulcer the patient is instructed to apply cotton swabs or gauze soaked in an iodiphore solution three or four times daily to cleanse an ulcer of bacteria and fungus.

Osteomyelitis

In medical practice another specialty is developing, the infectious disease specialist. I rely on his judgement in the selection and level of antibiotic required for many of my patients who have chronic bone infections. Figure 5 is the roentgenogram of the foot of a diabetic lady in her 50s. For two years she has

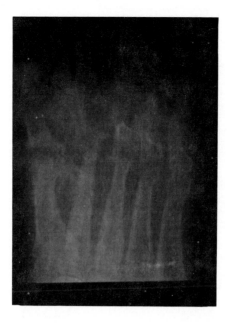

Figure 5.

had two draining sinuses on the sole of her foot associated with osteomyelitis of the first and second metatarsals and adjacent phalanges.

Both proper antibiotic and antibiotic serum level are required in order to be effective. The appropriate antibiotic and effective levels were determined after a piece of infected bone was sent to the microbiology laboratory and serum killing levels were measured against the chosen antibiotics. A resection of the first and second metatarsal or a ray resection of the first and second metatarsal was performed and a plantar flap was used to close the defect (Fig. 6). More important, the proper antibiotic was administered and her foot healed. The infectious disease specialist makes use of serum killing power. A patient's serum is used to culture the offending organism. Different levels of antibiotics are added to this serum. A level at which the antibiotic in serum effectively kills the bacteria is determined. This technique is valuable in assisting us with the correct level of antibiotics to be used in chronic osteomyelitis.

Metatarsal Phalangeal Dislocations

Few patients are seen with dislocations of the metatarsal phalangeal joint of the middle three rays and this dislocation may require an open reduction. In these cases usually the phalanx goes dorsal and the metatarsal goes dorsal to the metatarsal head. The volar plate that is firmly attached to the proximal phalanx

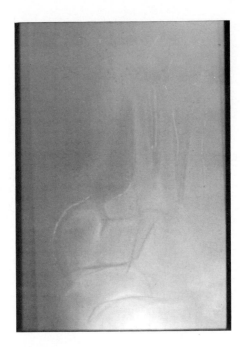

Figure 6.

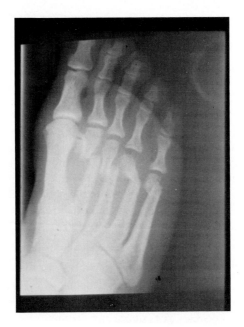

Figure 7.

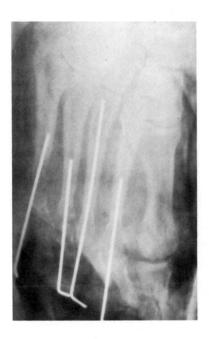

Figure 8.

on the plantar surface is displaced dorsal to the head of the metatarsal and prevents a closed reduction. A dorsal incision allows the operator to remove the lower plate from the joint and bring about the reduction.

Multiple Metatarsal Fractures

Internal fixation was utilized to stabilize the forefoot in this case (Fig. 7). The pale and cool toes promptly pinked up. The fracture healed. One should proceed with K wire fixation in this forefoot fracture as there was vascular insufficiency. Immobilization of the soft tissues resulting from secure fixation of the bones (Fig. 8) may allow better arterial and venous drainage. Power equipment, rheostats to control the speed of the drill, and a sterile environment are essential to carry out this procedure.

Questions and Comments

Moderator: William Trewartha

MODERATOR: Dr. Collett, are there any specific books that you recommend for study on diagnosis in pediatric development?

DR. COLLETT: There are several very good texts on growth and development. Probably the "grand-daddy" of them all was the one from Yale by Gazelle and Ilg, showing each stage of growth, from the newborn up to 16 years of age. I think "The Infant and Child in the Culture Today" is probably one of the best ones in the field. There are many more on the market but I highly recommend this particular text. This work gives a very good outline of normal physical and emotional child growth and development.

MODERATOR: Dr. Hawkins, what is the definition of an infectious disease specialist? Is he a bacteriologist or an M.D. who specializes in infections?

DR. HAWKINS: This man in medicine is a person who either has trained in pediatrics, and therefore by definition is a pediatrician or he is an internist dealing with infectious diseases in adult patients and thus becomes known as an internist or specialist in internal medicine. Therefore, he is a man who deals in either pediatrics or internal medicine. I am sure that in my own community the "infectious diseases man" is often a person who deals with chest problems and infections and thus becomes relegated to the responsibility of keeping his fellow physicians up-to-date on their antibiotics. There were several physicians on the pediatric service of the University of Colorado primarily involved with infectious diseases. Therefore, you have to check with your fellow pediatricians and internists to find out who among them are interested in these areas. Antibiotics are changing at such a rapid pace. You, like I, are burdened by the drug salesman who comes to you and says that: "this is the latest and the best," etc., etc. Under these circumstances, I frequently turn to the infectious disease specialist to advise me on the safety of the antibiotics concerned; and this is what I suggest you do also.

MODERATOR: Dr. Schuster, do you approve of the wedgie-type shoes?

DR. SCHUSTER: You will find that people who have to stand on their feet all day use the wedgie. If you look at the nurses, you will find that most end up wearing wedgies; waitresses and laborers too. Presently we have a rash of wooden-soled shoes, which, by the way, are excellent, for certain situations.

William Trewartha, D.P.M., *Denver, Colorado*

These in a sense are all wedgies — rigid shank shoes — and people gravitate to them because they are very comfortable to wear. I see no objection to them and I encourage them. People who work in a wet environment — bartenders, laundrymen — who wear ordinary shoes sometimes get their feet wet in the course of their job and the shoe thus tends to break down at the shank much faster. If you put a little wedge underneath those shanks, making them wedgies, they are much more comfortable.

MODERATOR: Another question for Dr. Schuster. Please comment on stretch socks and tight-fitting panty hose which have become popular these days.

DR. SCHUSTER: I think stretch socks could be very irritating and could result in some soft tissue damage. But I don't think stretch socks or panty hose could result in actual structural damage.

MODERATOR: This question is directed to Dr. Hawkins and concerns the usage of power equipment and placement of K wires. Do you place the K wire in the retrograde manner as you do with the hand drill?

DR. HAWKINS: This depends on whether the fracture is open or closed. If it is an open fracture, many times it is easier mechanically to place the wire distally out the sole of the foot and then retrograde it back. Obviously, if the fracture is closed and you are leaving it this way, thus reducing it and then internally fixing it, so therefore you cannot take an alternative step. But I must admit that with a hand drill it is difficult to insert a K wire without an open reduction of that and visualization of the fracture site. It depends on whether the fracture is an open or closed one.

MODERATOR: A question for Dr. Schuster. Medial or lateral sole wedging makes the sole rigid. Does this defeat the help derived from the wedgie?

DR. SCHUSTER: Medial and/or lateral sole wedging is fine for certain situations. The reason we would use a medial sole wedge on a shoe would be to stiffen the shoe on the medial side, also in order to act as a drag on the one side.

MODERATOR: Would each panelist please define his concept of the term "pronation"?

DR. HAWKINS: I consider this a problem which starts with position and think of it as something that is usually passive in the sense of examination. The subtalar joint in the hindfoot goes into a valgus position, and the forefoot into a position in which the first metatarsal ray is depressed more than the fifth metatarsal ray. The foot including the hind foot is in what I call a pronated position.

DR. COLLETT: As a pediatrician, I don't go in for all of the fancy terms. I see the child's foot as it is. For example: a child is standing on one foot, I can see the sole, there is a perfectly good arch. Then, when weight-bearing is applied, the whole arch collapses, the result to me is pronation.

DR. SCHUSTER: I am going to duck this question a little bit and repeat Dr. Inman's idea. Nature doesn't care much how one walks as long as he gets from 'here' to 'there' with maximum efficiency." I happen to agree with that. I assume we are discussing abnormal pronation. What bothers me about pronation is that we have averages to go by, but there doesn't seem to be a standard. I think everyone on this panel will agree that we can have feet that are really pronated according to the textbook and yet function beautifully.

DR. ROOT: Pronation is a motion, abduction, eversion and dorsiflection of the foot at the subtalar joint in an open change state in which the foot is non-weight bearing. When the foot is weight-bearing, we find that the calcaneus everts, the talus abducts and the plantarflexes on the calcaneus and that is pronation. It has nothing to do with pathology per se. Excessive pronation or pronation at the wrong time is pathological. The height of an arch has nothing to do with pronation. A foot with a varus calcaneus is normal in utero but if it is not outgrown by the time the child learns to walk and is inverted relative to the flood when it pronates to its maximum, it may still be slightly inverted as far as the calcaneus is concerned, or vertical. It may not show the evidence of pronation to the untrained eye. But the latter is clear in the instability of the forefoot and the foot will be traumatized. You will develop bunions, hammer toes and callouses and apparently still have a good arch foot. The height of the arch is unimportant and unrelated to the degree of pronation which occurs in the foot.

MODERATOR: Dr. Collett, how do you differentiate between an ataxic cerebral palsy and a Charcot-Marie-Tooth syndrome when the patient presents a pes cavus foot and claw toes?

DR. COLLETT: Cerebral palsy is usually an acquired condition from some cerebral damage, either a history of anoxia, birth trauma — some factor that has actually damaged the brain. The Charcot-Marie-Tooth is of course a hereditary condition that is progressive. There is evidence of the pathology later in the child's life and degeneration takes place. The cerebral palsy shows up fairly early as the child grows. The pes cavus and the cerebral palsy are later developments as they are actually weight-bearing. The other condition comes on considerably later when the actual diagnosis has been made.

MODERATOR: Dr. Root, please discuss hyperextension of the knees combined with knock-knees in pronation? Does the hyperextended knee change the approach towards treatment?

DR. ROOT: Hyperextension of the knee occurs in early childhood when the superior plateau of the tibia is tilted posteriorally. If we are dealing with an internal femoral torsion, we will find in either case that the knee may hyperextend in compensation for these particular deformities. The knee subluxes posteriorly and slides off the superior surface of the head of the tibia. As a result, we have what is referred to as a genu recurvatum. Normally a genu recurvatum would reduce as the person becomes older but it may not disappear completely, contrary to what Luther Davies in England said. We see many cases in which it stays. We still see the genu recurvatum at the knee in the adult. When you have the person stand with his feet in a neutral position, when the feet are pronated, it tends to unlock the knee and he stands in a slightly flexed or vertical position. But the deformity is still present. It may be masked by a compensated position.

Genu valgum is a position which may develop from the hip or distally from the foot. If the hip is in a proxi vari position it will mean that the midline of the shaft of the femur will be directed toward the opposite femur and will result in a genu valgum originating proximally. Take a person who is pronating abnormally, and pronating to maximum, particularly at the stance phase of gait, and at the contact phase, where he is carrying his foot in a maximum position of pronation throughout swing, and it strikes the floor in a maximum position of pronation — there is no eversion of the calcaneus left. The eversion force which is directed against the calcaneus (since it can't move it) will be reflected up the limb and a pronated foot unlocks the knee. So that you have a hypermobile knee in any person who is maximally pronated. Therefore, the first point of subluxation which can occur is at the knee. We will then find the tibial valgum developing as a result of the eversion force directed through the calcaneus and up through the tibia to the knee.

MODERATOR: Dr. Schuster, please comment on the hip-carrying position that many mothers use to transport their children strapped to the side of their mother.

DR. SCHUSTER: I can't see any harm in this. Hip-straddling spreads the legs. Legs can be spread by clothing, too — diapers, snowsuits, and other apparel. This has a definite effect on the way an individual walks. The more a youngster's feet are spread apart (their width of stance is probably 6-8 inches when they first start), the more out-toed he becomes. This sometimes becomes a source of concern to the parents but in itself is not really important.

DR. HAWKINS: You are not talking about foot deformity that would result from this, but are instead referring to the position of the hip. You ask: Is that a good position for the hip to be in? It certainly is! I think most of you know that the highest incidence of congenital dislocations of the hip is among the Indian tribes of the Southwest U.S.A. where children are strapped on carrying boards. You will find that if the child is allowed to straddle the back or the hip, the hips are brought out into abduction. This is a position where the femoral head is deeply seated in the acetabulum and considered to be the favorable position for rest in the newborn and young infants.

I would like to ask Dr. Schuster if we can move over to discussion of the fracture of the fifth metatarsal. It is a well-known fact that people who injure their ankles and who have other fractures, always give a history that is notoriously inadequate. The patient has no real recollection of exactly what happened to his foot when he injured it. I have never been able to elicit from the patient enough information for me to evaluate it as an avulsion fracture. It is usually transverse, as most of you know, but I am not sure if it is a direct blow to the side of the foot — the patient usually says that he inverted his foot — or whether it is, instead, an avulsion injury. I didn't quite catch what Dr. Schuster said about supporting the shoe in order to prevent such a fracture and I would like him to elucidate further.

DR. SCHUSTER: I believe I gave the wrong impression! I mentioned that it acts something like a judo chop. This gives you the false idea that it is a direct blow. The incidence of fractured fifths seems to be much higher with the use of flexible shank shoes. I can't comment on the evulsion aspect of it. Often patients do not realize that they have a fracture of the fifth — they cannot recall falling or anything like that. We are assuming this is so because they wear the special kind of shoe connected with this injury and we tie it in automatically with the high incidence of the fractured fifth. The treatment which is being used lately seems to work well. It consists of a rigid appliance that encompasses the plantar of the foot and the lateral side of the foot and acts as a very rigid shank. It can be of aluminum, steel, or any other material but it must be rigid; even fiberglass works.

DR. COLLETT: I want to make a comment here about mothers who carry their babies on their hip. It is not the children who have a problem, it is the mothers. The latter can get quite a bit of scoliosis and abnormal posture from this position. But — being a pediatrician, I can hardly be the one who should point that out!

DR. ROOT: A comment on supinatory sprain of the foot. The midtarsal joint has a range of motion in which it will not allow for supinatory compensation. That is, when the subtalar joint is in a neutral position in a normal foot, that would be with the calcaneus vertical to the floor — the normal foot in extremity. We have a situation in which the forefoot is locked relative to the rearfoot at the midtarsal joint. So the forefoot will not evert any further than is parallel with the plantar surface of the rearfoot. Therefore the forefoot and the rearfoot are on the same plane parallel to the floor and the forefoot cannot evert from this position. Now carry this foot into an inverted rearfoot position. The forefoot is locked so that it must also go into inversion with the rearfoot. As opposed to a pronated or everted position of the calcaneus, the forefoot has the ability to supinate and compensate in the metatarsal joints so it stays with the flow of eversion of the calcaneus. But with calcaneal inversion the forefoot also inverts. This is when you fall to the outside, you have level instability with supination.

The styloid fracture, the cuboid subluxation, is a serious injury. It should always be checked, along with the supinatory ankle sprain, particularly if there is history of stepping into a hole or any other similar position where the forefoot is plantarflexed at the time of the injury. For instance, when walking down stairs tripping and coming down on the forefoot with all the body weight directed against the forefoot then the rearfoot inverts and the reactive force in the floor attempts to evert the forefoot which will not move — but it can dislocate or fracture. This is the reason for styloid fractures and is also responsible for severe subluxations between the cuboid and particularly the fourth and fifth rays — and occasionally between the cuboid and the calcaneus. The late Dr. Downey established radiographically, without question, that we could verify cuboid subluxation in this type of an injury on x-ray and this should be reduced by manipulation. It is one of the few cases where I think manipulation, immediate manipulation, is one of the most important treatments. If it isn't, this particular type of foot very often leads to disuse atrophy. Vascular necrosis is a serious problem in this type of foot as well as a pseudo post-traumatic type of atrophy.

MODERATOR: Dr. Hawkins, you mentioned that you will not speak of biomechanics but prefer to talk about surgery of the foot. From this I get the impression that you are separating these two areas. If this is true, how do you justify this theory?

DR. HAWKINS: It is certainly not true. I think that we established earlier in the lectures that biomechanics is an investigation of the normal motions of the foot and is not directed at this stage towards totally correcting all problems. I am sure that we all recognize this. I did not wish to imply that I am not interested in biomechanics of the foot or that I am not willing to discuss the subject. I like biomechanics.

DR. ROOT: This is one time when I must take exception to Dr. Hawkins. I think that the future of surgery in the foot will be based upon biomechanics. You have to understand the full patho-mechanical development of the bunion which starts at about 3½ years of age. I recommend you to studies on the unshod foot where we find hallux abducto valgus deformity forming in unshod populations, regardless of foot gear. The deformities are just as great.

We have pictures in our office of natives in Africa who have never had shoes on in their lives and who developed bunions as large as any we see. Their feet are not irritated by a shoe and they may not hurt but nevertheless they have these deformities. In our society they would produce pain. Foot gear is a necessary evil in our culture. We are dealing with a situation in which the various aspects of biomechanics leading to the development of hallux abducto valgus are just now being understood. What is obvious is that there is no single suitable procedure for hallux abducto valgus surgery. Each case has to be studied according to the mechanical difficulty which is producing the problem. If you don't do something about the cause, you can anticipate a poor result postoperatively, perhaps even quickly, as in an equinus; or, over a longer time, as in forefoot varus. Forefoot valgus produces a prompt failure in bunion surgery. We can relate this to hammer toe surgery. Some hammer toes and clawtoes are related to the angle of the adductus of the forefoot, others to the abnormal mechanics of the quadratus plantae, and still others to just a single long digit. Until you begin to evaluate cause and effect, therefore, how can you determine a specific procedure to handle these defects and prognosticate what your result is going to be? I don't think it can be done and it hasn't been done in the past. I trust that in future we start progressing to the stage where we can determine in advance what we can anticipate and what needs to be done for a certain foot postoperatively.

DR. HAWKINS: We will need many more podiatrists and physicians in order to educate the public to reach this level of sophistication. I am a busy orthopedist. Dr. Collett is a busy pediatrician. We find it difficult, from day to day, to keep up with existing problems. I think that what is proposed eventually for the people and companies with the necessary funds will be screening clinics in which the podiatrist will inevitably be involved. His notions about biomechanics and their relationship to chronic foot problems will have to become much better known than they are now. You have a big job ahead of you. It is a reasonable one. But it is going to take a great deal of education, many more doctors and podiatrists, and more enlightened people. Too often I see a patient who presents himself routinely in the clinic who has a permanent foot deformity. I think all of us would agree that in this case it is difficult to restore the foot once more to its normal condition. So we have a real job on our hands! Taking into account the way preventive medicine is coming to the forefront in this country, I think that in the years to come, Dr. Root will be able to fully implement his ideas. I see it as a great and responsible assignment.

MODERATOR: Dr. Root, what foot conditions have given you the greatest failure rate in treatment with finished appliances?

DR. ROOT: Without question, any equinus or condition in which the foot cannot be dorsiflexed to 10 degrees with the subtalar joint neutral and the knee extended, is going to produce problems. If this foot has an acquired shortage of the gastroc-soleus which is very common, it will stretch out. But if there is the classical functional adaptation picture of a medial flattening of a head of the talus, a wedging in the navicular, and a blank axis subluxation at the midtarsal joint, then this means that an equinus state was present during the early formative years of this child. We find this in cases when for some unknown reason during puberty the child suddenly outgrows the length of his musculature, temporarily, and then he catches up. At the present time we don't know what determines the rate of muscle growth as compared to bone growth. In some persons we discover that if they grow very rapidly then the bone will actually outgrow the musculature temporarily. For this reason we are reluctant to do anything surgically to children or teenagers in order to lengthen musculature restricting ankle joint motion until this state has been under observation for at least a year or two. Unless, of course, there are very positive congenital signs present on x-ray. The equinus is without question the most destructive of the common foot problems seen. We can't operate on a hammer toe fifth nor on any of the forefoot lesions and anticipate a prolonged result in the presence of an equinus. Furthermore, we can do nothing to control function of the foot in the presence of an equinus. We can relieve sprain by casting the foot in a pronated position and reduce some postural fatigue. But we can do nothing about the lesions, the progress of the hallux abducto valgus deformity or the hammer toes.

Any surgery that we embark upon should be done only for extreme pain because this generally results in further complications and a need for even more surgery. I also include here all metatarsal head resection, or plantar keratomas in which, over a period of time, the patients can again develop a callous under the stump of the second metatarsal. I have seen this upon several occasions. That type of foot is a red flag whenever we see it. Any person with a congenital short hamstrings also develops equinus function. He has a knee flex position in locomotion and, therefore, requires more ankle joint motion than normal. If he has a normal ankle joint, then he needs pronation in the subtalar joint and subluxation in the metatarsal joint to get the added dorsiflection, which does not occur at the ankle. In this particular case surgery is also a failure. All the other defects which we recognize at present respond very well to care, some better than others. For instance, a forefoot valgus is a propulsive phase deformity and rearfoot varus is a contact phase deformity. The latter is more difficult to control than the former, but fortunately produces less symptomatology. As a result of this, even though we aren't controlling the foot by 100% at all, if we can get 50 or 60% improvement in function, this is usually enough to relieve symptomatology, avoid progressive deformity and also prevent future major surgery.

DR. SCHUSTER: I would like to hear Dr. Root elaborate his methods of preventing excessive pronation.

DR. ROOT: Control is accomplished through a lightweight acrylic appliance. You can see this type on display at the Burns Orthopedic Laboratory booth. We use first the shell which is the basic acrylic orthotic itself. We take a neutral position cast of the subtalar joint where the foot is neither pronated nor supinated and the midtarsal joint is locked in full pronation. In the normal foot that would be a parallelism between the plantar plane and the forefoot, and the plantar plane and the rearfoot. If you have a forefoot varus deformity — when you take a cast then you will find that the forefoot would be inverted. In a forefoot valgus, it would be everted. These defects must be supported degree by degree, otherwise they will set up a retrograde force which will pass back to the rearfoot and force abnormal motion. For example, if you have a plantar-flexed first ray, then you are going to have a pronatory abnormality and you have a supinatory compensation, which first appears in the midtarsal joint and then later on in the subtalar joint. If this happens to be a congenital plantar flexed first ray, you have the etiology of a shapeless foot. It is not contractured soft tissue, which is the result of position, and it is not a causative factor for these problems. When you do a wedge osteotomy and bring the first ray back to a normal position, all the soft tissue contracture stretches out and you see that the claw toe has disappeared and the toes straighten out. This type of deformity accompanies most equinus club feet. I find beautiful surgery done for the equinus element but nobody looks at the forefoot for the plantarflexed first ray. Thus, a lateral instability develops with pain at the ankle joint postoperatively. In many instances, we have to go ahead and do a wedge osteotomy in order to prevent this problem.

We need to support the defect in order to be able to control function. The basic acrylic shell itself has a round bottom. The inferior surface is not flat and, therefore, we must then wedge the rearfoot into its neutral position. If we have an 8 degree varus of the calcaneus, we would have to invert the heel by 8 degrees in heel strike in order to get that foot to the neutral position to eliminate the pronation. We can't do that with a shoe wedge because this type has a flat plane in the shoe and the foot slides off. It immobilizes the foot if you have a good solid heel counter, but when the heel counter breaks down, the wedge doesn't affect the position of the calcaneus at all. With the round bottom appliance we now have a wedge specifically applied to the soft tissue contour of the heel. We can now control the heel contact position. Also, we grind that, so that the appliance will evert with the foot, allowing the calcaneus to evert also by going under the exact number of degrees we wish. Generally, we allow for 6 degrees which is the average range which we found on the biomechanical charts that you see. This is for feet that appear to function efficiently. We will need to support the forefoot defects, then, by either adding plaster to the cast and supporting it in the appliance itself or by what we call forefoot posting. This is wedging the forefoot of the appliance to bring the floor up to meet the foot, so it doesn't fall back to produce forefoot pronation or supination.

DR. SCHUSTER: I understood Dr. Hawkins wanted to know how you handle a foot that pronates because of a short heel cord? However, I would like to let that hang fire for a minute. I shall comment on Dr. Root's advice. I was in thorough approval when he said that we should "wait and see." We must take a definitely conservative attitude toward heel cord lengthening. While we are doing a rash of heel cord lengthenings I am not sure the results justify them. Before we get involved with calf-muscle lengthening, I suggest that we had better find out what causes it, in the first place.

Dr. Root made several suggestions and I think he left the door open for other ideas. One of the possible answers to this problem is that we have to realize that man may be developing off his foot. Trying to treat pronation with a short heel cord is like rowing a boat that is tied to the dock! It can't be done. Do you lengthen the heel cord or do you adapt to it? I don't try to stretch heel cords any more. I am not ashamed to admit that I adapt to it and am sure that my patients are much happier. I raise the heel because I am satisfied in my own mind that this is the way to tackle most of these problems.

DR. ROOT: Lengthening the heel cord for an equinus problem is a serious undertaking. If you lengthen a muscle that is short because of a contracture state, it has the ability to be stretched back to its normal physiological length unless it is unfortunately spastic. If you have chronic spasm you have to find the etiology from a proprioceptive standpoint in the foot or in the extremity. If you are dealing with a clonic spasm, look for upper motor neuron lesion; and, if tonic, look for lower proprioceptive problem. It is necessary to rule these out. Dr. Trainer at St. Mary's Hospital has done multiple procedures on C.P.'s in which there are spastic gastrocsoleus, a spastic posterior tibial and spastic flexors; long and short flexors of the toes. As much as 1½" of the Achilles tendon is removed, plus a resection of the posterior tibial plus all flexors to the digits. Eighteen months later, however, they have to do the procedure over again because of reattachment. This procedure is ineffective for spastic cases.

The only lengthening that I can recommend is the congenital short gastric nemias where there is a normal ankle joint range when the knee is flexed and the subtalar joint is neutral. This is the *only* instance when it should be done and then *only* if there is evidence on bone of congenital presence that existed when the child first began to walk and develop. Loss of inclination angle of the calcaneus — practically a rocker bottom type of foot — which results from a midtarsal joint subluxation, must be there before one can assume a congenital deformity. I see all kinds of tendon-achilles lengthenings for patients who have not been able to adequately control function because of poor technique or diagnostic ability. This, however, is no excuse for performing surgery.

MODERATOR: Dr. Collett, does anemia in children show specific pathological findings? What would be the manifestations?

DR. COLLETT: Anemia causes considerable pathological manifestations in children. There are various types of anemia, including iron deficiency anemia, where there is lack of ingestion of iron; hemolytic anemias which cause problems with debilitation — resulting in lack of active movement, for instance. The general health of the child is then not good and he is more susceptible to infections. Therefore, any time anemia is found in the child it should be promptly treated. I think it is important to find the cause of the anemia first of all, and determine the degree of hemoglobin production, the areas of hemanophoresis where the blood is manufactured.

DR. ROOT: One of the manifestations of iron deficiency anemia in the foot is rheumatic inflammatory disease in which there is periarticular swelling, particularly the metatarsal phalangeal joints and periosteal inflammation on the lateral and medial sides of the calcaneus. There is also Achilles tendonitis and periosteal inflammation along the shaft of the fifth metatarsal, which is sufficiently superficial so that you can copy it. We have seen several instances in adults as well as in children. The moment that the anemia was treated the symptoms disappeared. There are many cases that we are overlooking in our profession — systemic conditions such as urinary tract and bladder infections, which are producing identical rheumatic inflammatory processes in adults. This condition is very common in children. Dr. Collett informed me that in the prepuberty period — in young girls particularly — urethritis and bladder infections are quite common and not reducible by medication but by dilation only. It needs someone to recognize these symptoms and who takes them seriously enough to treat the problem. Unfortunately, one of the situations that the podiatrist has to bear with for the time being until better communications with general medicine are established is the fact that when he recognizes rheumatic inflammatory process in the foot and needs further investigation of the systemic problems of this patient, it is not severe enough in the eyes of the internist or the pediatrician or the physician to warrant further investigation that is so often sorely necessary. The medical doctor doesn't look at foot problems, or consider them to be sufficiently serious. Somehow, we have to educate medicine before we can ever attempt to educate the public to the fact that these symptoms are the first signs of systemic disease. We are not physicians of the foot — at least I am not. I need medicine, every specialty in medicine! But when I refer a case to a medical doctor, I only wish that he would take it a little more seriously even though it is just "a foot problem."

MODERATOR: Dr. Root, please discuss the biomechanics and pathomechanics of stress fractures — multiple or single.

DR. ROOT: A stress fracture is nothing more than a fatigue of the bone which may occur from excessive usage. Even normal bone can fracture. For instance, we see this in the calcaneus and in the metatarsus in the military with boys who haven't been used to walking 25 miles per day. They take a long hike with a fairly heavy load and the first thing you know, they have a stress fracture. But most of what we see in our practice is not related to excessive activity at all, but instead to an intrinsic factor within the bone or the biomechanics of the foot itself. First of all, rheumatoid arthritis and some of the other systemic diseases produce a considerable degree of demineralization of bone which thus weakens it. If a loss of cortex substance is great, the bone is more apt to be fractured. Secondly, should the hallux not be able to function as a propulsive organ and weight must be transferred to the metatarsus — which are not normally propulsive organs to any extent, then we are consequently overloading the metatarsus. Cases of successive fractures of the metatarsus are not uncommon in the person who has rheumatoid arthritis, particularly when the subtalar joint is involved. Because it is painful to move the foot into a neutral position or supinatory position, the patient walks with his foot pronated. This tends to free the first ray and make it hypermobile so that the hallux cannot function as a propulsive organ. It becomes apparent that there is subperiosteal activity in the plantar nodules and, in many cases, fatigue fractures develop in this area.

I would like to caution those of us who like to do neuroma surgery. The fact is, most of the neuroma surgery done is quite unnecessary. When you recognize rheumatic inflammatory processes, you will eliminate 95% of neuroma surgery. The neuroma has a specific history which should be carefully taken before the diagnosis of neuroma is made. I do not see how a mistake can be made if the patient is evaluated properly. We have many cases of Raynaud's disease and Raynaud's phenomenon which are operated upon for neuromas. I have seen five neuroma surgeries performed in five years, not only by podiatrists but also by orthopedists on the same patient who actually had nothing more than Raynaud's disease! This is the sort of thing that I think is happening throughout medicine today. Incompatible diagnosis is being made of the foot. One of the benefits of biomechanics is that it enables us to study joints for fluid, for abnormal quality of motion and it immediately tells us whether or not we are dealing with systemic disease. We may not find the etiology. But we must pursue it. The mechanical trauma that affects the foot is seldom, if ever, so acutely painful that the person cannot bear weight on the foot. When you have acute inflammatory process in the foot, think proximally.

DR. HAWKINS: Dr. Schuster, you talked about positional problems in children. I cannot disagree with anything that you said. But what I would like to ask is: how do you do it? Usually I try to educate the mother to keep her child from sitting on his feet. Also, you didn't mention problems involved when sleeping? Some children drag their feet up under them when asleep and may continue the problem of tibial torsion during their napping or night hours.

DR. SCHUSTER: Certainly, if a child has unusual sleeping habits, I tell the mother not to bind this child down in bed with a blanket. Let him be free. About the television watching habit: I think I have already mentioned that you should try to discourage the child from sitting in this manner. I am sure, Dr. Hawkins, that you will agree that it is a pretty tough goal to try to inculcate a certain habit in children! You can't get them to do exercises. All you can do is talk to them and try to impress the parents with the importance of changing the child's sitting habits.

DR. ROOT: A curious thing. If you will look at Japanese culture and the manner in which they sit on their feet — and realize they have done so from earliest childhood right on through adulthood — why is it, then, that *they* don't develop torsional problems? We don't find any greater incidence of positional problems in those born and raised in Japan than we do in the Caucasian born and reared in this country. I don't believe that this position will alter anything more than soft tissue — and that only temporarily. The moment a person moves, the soft tissue automatically tightens right back up and he becomes normal. We have purposely had children sit on their haunches and on their feet watching television. I have measured them over a period of several years without seeing any significant change in measurements at either the hip or the subtalar joint or at any other joint in the lower extremity. I believe that people have made assumptions and those assumptions cannot be substantiated.

In dealing with torsion of the extremity, femoral torsion or tibial torsion, only ontogenesis is able to change the true torsion. If the torsional factor is not outgrown by the time the child is walking, it will continue until puberty. This is an interesting observation. Go through a high school, look at the freshman class and see how many cases of pigeon toes you have. Then look at the senior class and notice how many fewer cases of pigeon toe there is. How many pigeon toes do you see in the adult? But how many 10-11-12-13 year-old children do you see with pigeon toes? During puberty there is a rapid reduction. I had the opportunity to observe 1,700 children in the San Luis Obispo schools. And I saw these changes myself. They were unrelated to any treatment and are normal torsional development. The only procedure necessary is to protect the foot so that it doesn't pony abnormally during the time the torsion is reducing. Once the torsion is reduced you can take the orthotic off. It is not needed any further, providing, of course, that there is no serious foot defect. In dealing with rotational abnormalities of the hip, muscular abnormalities or neuromuscular disease you will find a difference in the range and symmetry of range of motion from one side to the other. Particularly, you will discover a variance between a hip-flexed and a hip-extended positon when you rotate. This is why measurements are so important. They are vital for us to begin to unravel some of the fact from fiction. We are dealing more with fiction in the lower extremity than we are with fact!

Davis' Law, published in 1857 in the American Medical monthly magazine, is still being quoted; and is still being taught in podiatry school, "soft tissue will respond to stretching." Tissue will respond *only* if it is in a contracture state, and under certain circumstances. If there is a chronic spasm, it is going to shorten up again. It is necessary for us to begin to develop a better scientific basis for what we do and what we believe.

DR. HAWKINS: I heartily second what Dr. Root says. I may be interpreting my own feelings, however, I do not think we should first try to convince the physicians. Every branch of medicine has developed from the members of its own society. If you want to develop special fields of interest, you cannot say, "We are going to be general physicians." Dr. Collett showed children's feet and he mentioned some of the mucopolysaccharidosis in the hands today. Dr. Bob Horner who is a hand surgeon here in Denver is trying to delineate changes in the hands of children with mucopolysaccharidosis. Learn biomechanics and be well-based in the basic sciences so necessary for the practice of podiatry. It is a wrong idea to consider joining with medicine for we don't really have any thing to offer. It is *you* people who will have something to offer to *us*. I think we can get along very well just as we are. Most subspecialities in medicine have grown just because someone became interested in a certain area of medicine and he pursued his interest. I don't think there is a really big battle going on at all.

DR. COLLETT: To summarize: I have learned a lot more from you people than I feel you have learned from me! I feel that further communications between the specialists of podiatry and certainly pediatrics and internal medicine should be developed considerably and that we should all work together for the good of our patients.

II. Emerging Trends in Health Care — A Challenge to Private Practice

National Health Insurance

Emmett G. Zerr, Jr.

Before I speak to the general subject of "Emerging Trends in Health Care" and my specific reflections on National Health Insurance, allow me to digress for a moment and speak of a gentleman, and a friend, who recognized the importance of involvement and community leadership as a part of his professional commitment.

I speak of the late Dr. C. A. Fritts, who was a member of the Colorado Health Planning Council, Chairman of its Legislative Committee, and a member of the Task Force on Prevention; a man who gave many hours of his valuable time to Comprehensive Health Planning in Colorado, and who most importantly gave strong professional leadership to a most ambitious planning effort. The example he has set for your profession is an envious one.

Much has been written on emerging trends in health care, and much has been written on National Health Insurance; however, my presentation will not concern itself with a difficult and perhaps boring summary or brief on what has been written.

Quoting from a speech given by Thomas J. Lupo, President, New Orleans Area Health Planning Council:

"While many of us recognize that aggressive efforts are required to improve the health of our nation, and most of us see health 'in crisis,' we must maintain cognizance that meeting the daily health needs of our nation is a complex and continual responsibility that cannot be allowed to falter. We cannot get so carried away that we allow a break in the essential continuity of that system. Our health system is deficient in many respects, particularly in its ability to meet the needs of many of our disadvantaged and indigent. It is still the best of the systems that man has been able to devise and the only one we have at the moment. We must correct our deficiencies and expand the system. In the meantime, however, the ongoing responsibility must not be allowed to fail through injudicious or simplistic efforts to rush into untried health delivery systems; or, by unfair, inaccurate, or intemperate criticism of *all* health

Emmett Zerr, *Executive Secretary, Colorado Comprehensive Health Planning Commission, Denver, Colorado.*

providers, in the vain hope that a particular plan will succeed. Above all, we cannot afford to tamper with the health of our people, motivated alone by political expediency."

I am not an expert on NHI and, therefore, cannot share all the ramifications of each bill; however, I am a health planner and, therefore, would like to share with you some of my observations as a professional, as well as those stated by a consumer in New Orleans on the necessity for an available, accessible health care delivery system that is both efficient and economical.

As a health planner, two things break out as the primary reason for the present thinking in terms of national health insurance, obviously in negative terms:

1. Medical care costs are rising to the point where people in all classes cannot meet the expense of being ill, e.g., $100/day for a hospital room;

2. Many of the indigent, long recognized as a cachement for ill health, do not have health care available and accessible to them. Statistics bear this out.

"While we all recognize the urgent need to effect changes in our health care delivery system, we should not lose cognizance of the fact that some change is occurring, even though very slowly, and many changes will continue to occur through a great number of efforts, many of which involve support and participation by our nation's physicians, hospitals, and other health providers, with increasing involvement of consumers and our communities themselves."

Some of the specific bills for National Health Insurance are:

A. AMERIPLAN – Perloff report to the American Hospital Association.
B. PELL – Minimum health benefits and health services distribution and education act.
C. KENNEDY– Health security act.
D. JAVITS – National health insurance and health services improvement act.
E. GRIFFITHS – National health insurance act.
F. A.M.A. "MEDICREDIT" – Health insurance assistance act.
G. BURLESON – National health care act.
H. NIXON – National health insurance standards act (for employers); Family health insurance (for poor)

I feel compelled to inform you that in all of the legislation I have read that is in current discussion and debate in our nation concerning this matter, nowhere have I found yet the type of thrust or commitment that I personally believe is necessary to bring about those changes that are needed in the system.

In my humble judgment, most of the legislation still places priority upon treatment for poor health with considerable emphasis on facilities. In none of them have I found the type of massive fiscal support at any level, toward research, education, manpower development, use of technological advances in other fields, corporate systems, management concepts, accessibility, accountability, all of which I think are the necessary ingredients and must have super priority if we are to change the system, one of basically the treatment of disease, to a system designed for the delivery of health.

I get no consolation, nor does any American, from a system which assures me that I can 'die comfortably and painlessly in an excellently structured, aesthetically pleasing, sanitary facility of my choice from the dreaded disease of cancer.'

I, like any other American, want a system that can give me some assurance that I can 'live in health' without the fear of cancer.

It would behoove us all to recognize that in today's society, it is an accepted fact that health is a 'right' for every citizen in this nation, carrying with it the normal complement of responsibilities – but nevertheless 'a right.'

If we are going to make this right 'accessible and functional' in the 70's, all of us in our consideration of pending legislation should put aside our selfish interest, discontinue any thrusts which might be interpreted as obstructionism, roll up our sleeves, join together and buckle down and constructively propose alternates that in our judgment can assist in delivering 'this right' and, at the same time, adjust our selfish interests to be compatible with a program for health that each citizen of this nation deserves.

The question we should ask ourselves is how our discipline can be adjusted, expanded, improved, to fit into an expanded and improved system of the type required to deliver health to this nation's citizens.

How long must we consider as the obstructionist view that this or that piece of legislation further tears down the 'patient-doctor relationship,' or the right of the patient to select a particular doctor??? Nowhere, however, have I heard any thrust that would take the 800,000 indigents that walk through the Charity Hospital in New Orleans who have *no* choice of doctors, who have *no* doctor-patient relationship – nowhere do I hear any thrust to provide for these better than a million people each year this so-called patient-doctor relationship, this so-called right of choice – in times of emergency, in times of accident, find ourselves in that same Charity Hospital, or in another similar institution or proprietary institution, getting emergency care from expert providers who have no so-called doctor-patient relationships with us, and who are not necessarily doctors of our choice, but who under these conditions provide for us the type of expertise and attention that in many cases saves our lives, or keeps us alive until such time as we are in a position 'only through out affluency' to provide this 'patient-doctor relationship' and right of choice.

Please do not misinterpret this remark in any way to conclude that I am opposed to the right of any citizen to select his own doctor. What I am saying is that a vast majority of the consumers of this nation *do not now have that right.*

If it is determined that the system we are attempting to develop should provide that right, it should provide it for *all*, not just those of us who are affluent enough to afford it.

In no legislation in the public forum today have I observed a thrust for 'accountability' in situations of this type, nor is there the fiscal support available to create consortiums of the type that might jointly deliver these services to many independent institutions on a basis affecting vast economic savings to the consumer and the provider.

I personally find it incomprehensible that I can sit at my television set and see the technology of this nation provide the opportunity to view, communicate with, and protect our men in space as far away as the moon; to observe our control of man's environment in space; to listen to his very heartbeat, evaluate his pulse, temperature, and even anticipate and adjust for his potential temporary illness, and yet stand by on this planet and not be knowledgeable of either the conditions, diagnosis, symptoms, or desires of the indigent people within a few miles of some of the best health care facilities in the nation.

I can find no satisfaction in the great storehouse of knowledge that a person like myself can acquire through the television media and become almost an 'arm-chair' expert in space through this communication media – yet find that it has been so sparsely utilized in the field of health that many of our people don't even know where, how, or what health care and treatment is available to them, nor is there broad knowledge of what they should do to maintain and conserve their health.

Unfortunately, in all of the legislation I have read, nowhere do I find priority or massive fiscal support for the type of educational process for our children, adults, and potential mothers, in the fields of family planning, the conceptual process, and human behavior that in my judgment could lead this nation to conceive and bring forth a new generation of healthy beings.

Nowhere have I found serious commitment to bring the facilities and multidisciplinary provider groups to the people to be served. I find instead continued priority to improving the existing facility.

Nowhere have I found the type of fiscal thrust necessary to provide the opportunity to make some form of medical provider out of indigent, unemployed, consumers who represent a vast part of our national health problem. It is *not* my intention in these latter observations to be critical of any of those involved in either the planning for, or delivery of health in this nation, but only to add my one small voice to encourage us to work together, to plan together, to propose together, that type of affirmative, positive, action which deep in each of your consciences you know is necessary if the citizens of this nation are to receive their 'right to health' in the 70's.

In Colorado, the Colorado Health Planning Council, which is a consortium of consumers and providers, feels that any respectable system for delivery of health services should include a component of education, recognition of the role that environment plays on a person's health, planning for health care systems that provide for the delivery of acute and chronic care, and last, but perhaps most important, that area of preventing ill health.

At this time in the history of our nation, there is no room for intemperate or articulate rhetoric, nor is there room for playing the political numbers game. Neither rhetoric, nor politics can contribute to the adjustment of our health delivery system to that level which the conscience of this nation demands. The opportunities at this moment in our history are inestimable; — the challenge is great — the future to be gained is unlimited; however, those of us who are too timid, too self-serving, too negative and are not bold, imaginative or daring enough to adjust to this challenge, will have no future.

Your role in the community process has been defined by people like Dr. Fritts. Your input into what a National Health Insurance Plan should look like is important. I urge you to examine what has been proposed and express yourselves in what you feel best for people of our country through the American Podiatry Association and your Comprehensive Health Planning Council.

Health Maintenance Organizations

James L. Kurowski

Mr. Zerr has set a framework of events pertinent to the transition in health-care delivery systems. I would like to re-emphasize some of these. First, there are widespread differentials in health status among socio-economic groups in this country. To illustrate this, I can relate directly to my own experience as a county health officer in Mississippi. In Washington County the infant mortality rate was 50 per 1,000 live births; i.e., for every 1,000 children that were born, 50 would not reach their first birthday. The infant mortality for the black population in that area was 65 per 1,000 live births. For the whites, the rate was about 25 per 1,000 live births. At this time the national infant mortality was about 25 per 1,000 live births. It doesn't take a statistician to recognize that these are widespread differentials and, furthermore, that access to medical care could alleviate much of this differential. I realize that for many of you who practice entirely in suburban areas and on middle class patients, it is difficult to conceive of these differentials. Let me assure you they are real.

While there are these differentials, there has also been a change over time in the mortality and morbidity patterns of the non-poverty population which should be considered in prescribing a direction to improve the organization for health care delivery. The majority of our population now suffers from chronic diseases. Fifty years ago the principal cause of death was tuberculosis. Other infectious diseases also ranked high. Now the principal causes of death are arteriosclerotic heart disease, cancer, and other chronic conditions which require a long-term management. These conditions are not easily modified by short-term intervention but require continuous management, and in many instances, a change in the life-style of the patient.

The second point from Mr. Zerr's statement which I wish to emphasize is the increase in health expenditures. National health expenditures rose from $12 billion in 1950, to $67 billion in 1970. Estimates of expenditures for 1975 run to $110 & $120 billion dollars. Is it any wonder that government is becoming increasingly interested in what is being bought for those amounts of money?

James L. Kurowski, M.D., *Assistant Professor School of Medicine, Department of Preventive Medicine and Comprehensive Health Care, University of Colorado Medical Center, Denver, Colorado.*

A third set of events is the advance in knowledge and technology in the health field, e.g., there are new and improved immunization techniques for polio, measles, mumps, as well as dramatic breakthrough in organ transplants. However, the most significant events affecting delivery of care may not be in the bio-medical sciences but in the communications industry. This technology is likely to alter professional practice patterns considerably. It will be possible to better monitor the encounter of a professional with a patient and to better evaluate its outcome and what is being paid for.

I would make one last observation. It is quite amazing that despite the wide variations among the national health insurance proposals, there is an element of consensus. Most recognize the need to bring some order, some organization, some new incentives to the delivery of health care. Whether we call that approach a Health Maintenance Organization as the Administration does; or Comprehensive Health Services Organizations, as the Health Security Plan introduced by Senator Kennedy does; or whether we use the American Hospital Association term of Health Care Corporations; or Senator Pell's term of Health Services and Health Education Corporations; we are talking about similar approaches to a recognized problem. There is a remarkable degree of consensus that there is a major problem in the organization and delivery of health care services.

With these four observations as background, let us examine the H.M.O. The objectives of the H.M.O. proposal are several. The first is to give the population, the consumers, a choice in the type of health care system it may utilize. It should be noted that this is not designed to provide a monolithic system of health care. It does not intend a replacement of existing traditional fee-for-service private practice system. Rather, the intent is to promote some alternatives to the existing system and these alternatives are believed to have certain advantages. The second objective is that of cost control, including incorporating incentives for the latter in the delivery system itself. The goal is to improve ability of Federal and State programs to control their health care expenditures by using prepaid contracts for its beneficiaries. The third objective is to provide incentives for health maintenance rather than for crisis-oriented care. The fourth and last objective is to use these incentive and investment funds to help correct some of the problems of maldistribution of health care services that exist in our country.

Having stated these objectives, let us proceed to a description of an H.M.O., (Health Maintenance Organization). According to the Administration, "a Health Maintenance Organization is based on four principles:

It is an organized system of health care which accepts the responsibility to provide or otherwise assure the delivery of
an agreed-upon set of comprehensive health maintenance and treatment services for

a voluntarily-enrolled group of persons in a geographic area and is reimbursed through a pre-negotiated and fixed periodic payment made by or on behalf of each person or family unit enrolled in the plan." Each of these principles should be elaborated upon.

An *organized system of health care* is one that arranges for the provision of services of physicians and other health professionals, the services of inpatient and outpatient facilities for preventive, acute, and rehabilitative care, for their defined population in a systematic fashion. It promises continuity of care for the enrolled population through linkages between components of the system. It should be recognized that these promises are relative.

Comprehensive health maintenance and treatment services mean that the H.M.O. is capable of providing for a range of services including primary care, emergency care, acute inpatient hospital and rehabilitative care.

Some populations may be able to purchase from the H.M.O. the entire range of health services, including primary care, emergency care, inpatient hospital care, as well as dental, podiatric and other needed health care. Most population groups will purchase something less than this full range of services from the health maintenance organization. As a minimum, it is likely that the Government regulations will insist that they should be able to provide either directly or arrange to pay for physicians' services, inpatient hospital care, and outpatient preventive medical services. In any case, even if the H.M.O. is not asked to provide all of the needed health services, it should at least be able to refer patients to qualified community resources. It should be noted that primary care is one of the keystones of the H.M.O. This may be more graphically described as "personal physician care" or the entry point into the system, from which referrals to specialists are guided.

An *agreed upon set of services* means that the consumers and the H.M.O. will agree upon which services will be purchased from the H.M.O. in return for the prepayment figure. Some H.M.O.'s may have groups of enrollees paid for by Medicare, or Medicaid, or by employer-employee arrangements and, therefore, the benefit schedules for population groups may differ.

The *enrolled group* means those individuals or groups of people who voluntarily join the H.M.O. through a contract arrangement in which the enrollee (or head of the household) agrees to pay the fixed monthly or other periodic payment (or have it paid on his behalf) to the H.M.O. The enrollee agrees to use the H.M.O. as his source of health care if he becomes ill or needs care. The contract is for a specified period of time (a year, for example).

The concept of the Health Maintenance Organization has been developed from the success of a variety of medical foundations and prepaid group practice organizations in various parts of the United States. These organizations are now providing health care services for some 7 million persons. The principles of these organizations have been extracted.

Thus, "Health Maintenance Organization" is an umbrella term which embraces a variety of types of health care systems. One can classify these systems along two dimensions: the relative degree of organization and centralization of health man power and facilities; and the exclusiveness of the facilities and professional groups' commitment to the enrolled population. That is, whether the facilities and professionals serve an enrolled population only, or combine an enrolled population with a fee-for-service population.

The most highly specialized and exclusively-committed model of the health organizations has multi-specialty physicians, and other health manpower, organized into a closed-panel group practice; it uses health facilities which are owned and operated by the organization. Both the group practice and the facilities are devoted entirely to serving the enrolled population groups on a full-time basis with minimal, if any, fee-for-service practice. This model is most closely identified with the Kaiser Foundation Health Plans and with the Group Health Cooperative of Puget Sound.

Lesser degrees of organization and exclusiveness of commitment are represented by H.M.O.'s which utilize either full or part-time physician group practices and have arrangements for the purchase of inpatient care with community health care facilities. The Health Insurance Plan of New York and the Group Health Association of Washington, D. C., represent this type of organization.

The least degree of centralization of organization and exclusiveness of commitment is represented by the foundations. These utilize individually practicing physicians and community health facilities. These units are bound together only by contractual and professional agreements and these serve an enrolled population side by side with a fee-for-service practice. The San Joaquin Foundation in California exemplifies this approach.

While the H.M.O. concept can embody any of these widely-differing health care systems, the organizations must accept the responsibility to deliver services (not just to pay for services), and assure that these are available to enrollees within the geographic service area on a 24-hour-a-day, 7-days-a-week basis. The H.M.O. must assure that each enrollee knows how and from whom services will be available. That is, there must be an effort made to assure appropriate entry point for each enrollee.

With this overview of the Health Maintenance Organizations concept, let us survey what the Department of HEW is doing to encourage the development of H.M.O.'s.

For most models of H.M.O.'s, the planning, the capital, and the initial operating costs are quite high. Thus, for the most highly organized and committed model of the Health Maintenance Organization, along the hospital-based group practice type, the estimates are that it takes upwards of 20,000 enrollees before the plan will break even. Planning costs can go as high as

$500,000. Operating deficits can amount to as much as $2 – $3 million. Capital investment costs and ambulatory care facilities can be in the range of $1 – $2 million, for a 20,000 member population.

To help meet these costs, the Administration has proposed a program of grants, contracts and loans, and loan guarantees, to provide incentive for groups to start these types of organizations.

The second part of the strategy is to provide for a Health Maintenance Organization option to consumers in public and private health insurance plans. Prepayment through the Health Maintenance Organization type arrangement is now being used in some state Medicaid programs. This option is being proposed under Medicare, in H.R. 1. This Bill was considered in the last session· of Congress as well. Furthermore, the health insurance industry *may be required* to offer an H.M.O. option to employee groups. An employee covered by an approved health insurance program would be able to choose to purchase care from either an H.M.O. or from the traditional health insurance program. It cannot go without saying, that there must be a Health Maintenance Organization in the area *where he lives* before he can ever have this choice.

While this package of proposals represents the future, the Department of H.E.W. is already supporting these Health Maintenance Organization developments under existing statutory authority. They are using authority under 314(e) Partnership for Health Program, and Research and Demonstration Authority from the National Center for Health Services Research and Development. In addition, they are developing a cadre of Federal personnel, as well as consultants in each region. These persons will provide technical assistance and advice in the development of Health Maintenance Organizations.

In conclusion, I will put before you some generic questions for our later discussions.

What implications do you see in this H.M.O. concept for podiatry?

Will podiatric practice differ in the future from its present patterns? If so, how might it differ? I only mention these now to stimulate your thinking.

REFERENCES

Myers, B. A.: Health Maintenance Organizations. Presented April 7, 1971, at the Annual Conference of State Comprehensive Health Planning Agencies, Washington, D.C.

Ellwood, P. M. Jr.: Impact on Providers & Delivery Systems. Presented November 12, 1970, at the National Health Insurance Conference, Philadelphia, Pennsylvania.

Bright, M.: Demographic Background for Programming for Chronic Diseases in the United States. *Chronic Diseases and Public Health*. Baltimore, Md., The Johns Hopkins Press, 1966, pp. 5-23.

Private Insurance Concepts in the Delivery and Financing of Health Care

James H. Hunt

Mr. Zerr said there wasn't room for rhetoric in this great national debate. One should not forget that universal law of politics – that when all is said and done, more is said than done.

Not long after President Kennedy was inaugurated, a reporter asked for his impressions of the first few months in office. He replied: "When we got into office, the thing that surprised me most was to find that things were just as bad as we'd been saying they were."

I've been with Aetna Life & Casualty almost two years. At the time I joined Aetna, I had a limited background in the technical aspects of health insurance and absolutely no experience with what is now known as the health care system, or nonsystem as the academicians love to call it.

The thing that has surprised me most in the months since I began studying this complex issue is that things are just about as bad in the delivery of medical services as the critics say they are.

We know that adequate medical services simply do not exist in many parts of our nation. We know of the very limited Medicaid benefits provided the poor in many states. We also understand that in other states – New York and California especially – those just above the Medicaid eligibility line are fed up at paying taxes so the poor can have better access to comprehensive medical care through Medicaid than the taxpayers do. We suffer silently when we hear of families afflicted with illnesses which devastate them financially, thinking that there, but for the grace of God or healthy parents or adequate nutrition or whatever, go I.

The problems demanding solution are almost endless. But similar problems afflict us in our efforts to deal with housing, with education, with our public services, etc. The less fortunate among us probably come off worse in those fields than in health care, even though the effects of decent housing, good

James H. Hunt, *Director, Government Relations, Group Division Aetna Life & Casualty, Hartford, Connecticut.*

nutrition, pollution-free cities, etc., upon health may be more important than a doctor next door.

It seems to me that what distinguishes health care as an issue from other compelling needs is very simply that costs are completely out of control. My own guess is that the independent, or middle-of-the-road, American adult who votes probably has reasonably good access to medical care and is not dissatisfied with the system. But when that same person reads about proposed Blue Cross rate increases of 20% to 30% and more, rate increases which bear no relationship to cost of living increases, he begins to wonder whether he's paying too much for his reasonable decent medical care. And when he hears that physicians' fees have gone up twice as fast as the cost of living in the last ten years while hospital charges have gone up four times as fast, he begins to wonder whether there isn't a better way. And his elected representative is listening.

And so, primarily as a result of the rampant inflation in medical care costs in recent years, health insurers now stand somewhere close to the edge of oblivion as the politicians respond to the cry for some solution, any solution, to the upward spiral in health care costs.

While there would be those who would argue that in the great march of history a program of national health insurance for everyone is in the cards as a matter of absolute inevitability, I think there is an equally good argument that, absent cost pressures of recent years, Medicare and Medicaid would now be more acceptable national programs responding to the needs of those which private carriers cannot reach, and that each could be expanded and improved to fill the gaps which still exist.

The inflation in medical care costs has hit commercial health insurers particularly hard because about 60% of the insurance dollar goes for hospital care. Some of the rate increases we and others have had to deliver to employers whose experience has been worse than average (and the averages are bad enough), have been very nearly unbelievable. Not a few employers are now asking themselves this reasonable question: "Could our employee health insurance plans result in more stable, predictable costs if an expanded Medicare, or the Kennedy program, or whatever, were enacted and financed through payroll taxes?" Thus, Thomas Watson of IBM now says that he supports such a solution as Kennedy's and admits such a thought would have been heresy 10 years ago.

So now the question for health insurers is no longer whether there *will be* national health insurance — Louis Harris poll last February found public support for a national health insurance plan to be 2 to 1 in favor and I find no one in my company or in the industry who thinks about the issue who believes there won't be — but rather whether the system of national health insurance which emerges from the legislative process will include a role for us and I mean a meaningful role, not just a bill-paying role under a giant Medicare program.

We are optimistic on this point.

In the first place, we believe most Congressmen believe that the health insurers have much expertise to contribute and are not as much a part of the problem as Senator Kennedy would have the public believe.

We are accused of not being able to control costs and of reaping profits from sickness. It's true that we can't control costs all by ourselves – we're not in the business of providing the services in the first place and, in the second place, our contracts bind us legally to pay bills as rendered in all situations except those involving outright fraud or abuse. Further, our clients, the employers we insure, want us to pay the employee's bills – otherwise they, the employers, would catch it from the employees or their labor unions.

As to the second charge – we're making lots of money – that's simply funny, at least for the largest insurers who write almost 60% of the industry's hospital and medical coverage. In the five years ending 12/31/70, these insurer's aggregate net losses were over a quarter of one percent of premiums. These are true losses and are not offset by any hidden gains from investment income.

The health insurance industry will survive, as Tom Wicker of the New York Times put it, only to the extent that we can contribute something to an effective workable national health program.

We believe we have contributed a great deal in the last 25 years to the good health of Americans. That we have not been able to do the whole job is no reason to be apologetic. In fact, we are proud of our accomplishments. As HEW Secretary Richardson says, the bottle is half full, not half empty. But we are not blind to the reality of the nation's health care problems.

It seems to me that the extent of the contribution the health insurance industry can make to an effective workable national health program depends directly on the extent to which that program incorporates a continuation of fee-for-service medicine. While we are normally thought of as risk takers, to a very large extent in the health insurance field the services we sell are our skills in managing reasonably efficiently the flow of paperwork that fee-for-service implies. The principal alternatives to a fee-for-service system – capitation payments to individual providers, health care institutions, or comprehensive health care organizations – has the effect, if you think about it, of transferring the risk to the provider. Further, there are no particular organizational skills involved in making lump-sum payments to providers based on the number of persons covered. Very simply, you don't need a middleman under the capitation payment principle.

The health insurance industry recognizes the obvious advantages which flow from capitation payments, especially to comprehensive health care organizations. Aside from the delivery advantages in an H.M.O. (Health Maintenance Organization) of continuity and comprehensiveness of care, centralized medical records, ease of referrals, etc., management of costs within the capitation payment concept is implicit: the individual or organization to whom such payments are made must live within a predetermined budget. Several large health insurers, including Aetna, are now working with medical groups and hospitals on an experimental basis to see if our organizational skills combined with marketing strengths can be employed profitably in developing prepaid group practices.

In considering what kind of national health insurance program to argue for, there is great appeal in going all the way with the capitation principle. The likelihood that such a national policy would pretty well eliminate health insurers, while alarming to those of us employed by health insurers, could be expected to be greeted with a great national yawn.

Nevertheless, despite the aggravating paperwork which fee-for-service implies, there is a great deal of flexibility to the system. It seems to me that few of the public are dissatisfied with fee-for-service per se and that many providers have a very large investment of money and careers in its continuation.

Thus, it seems to me that in the immediate future, fee-for-service will survive and so will health insurers. In the longer run, the survival of fee-for-service principle will be directly dependent upon containment of costs thereunder, as I see it.

I am reasonably optimistic that fee-for-service costs can be controlled, and that the rate of increase in health care costs from year-to-year that we have been experiencing can be reduced and brought into line with the consumer price index. Among the reasons I am optimistic are:

1. There has been considerable tightening up under the government programs of Medicare and Medicaid. For example, in 1970 Medicare spending increased 8% compared with 23% the previous year. Now proceeding through the Congress are further cost-tightening provisions in these programs.

2. Interest in medical care foundations, which are confined principally to the west coast, has been increasing rapidly in the last 18 months as doctors realize they must take steps to police their own practices if they don't wish to be on a government salary in the near future. The best of the foundation programs, at least in my opinion, include pre-admission certification for non-emergency hospital use. My understanding is that the medical care foundation in Sacramento County, California, has reduced hospital utilization about 20%.

3. Insurers are coming to the point of wanting more structured review mechanisms for private programs. We have been developing statistical profiles at Aetna for use in our group-health business.

4. There is quickening of interest in many states in seeking enactment of certificate-of-need legislation in order to combat the unneeded expansion of hospital and other health care institutions' facilities and services. There is also some interest being generated in putting hospitals under a kind of "public utility rate" regulation.

5. Doctors are beginning to speak as if they really might make peer review work, although I am exceedingly skeptical about this.

It occurs to me that years ago before the widespread development of third-party payment mechanisms, physicians used to treat their patients with a view toward the costs of such treatment in the case of those of modest income. By and large, the medical profession now is at the other extreme of the pendulum, exercising extremely little accountability for expenditures ordered on behalf of patients. It is not necessary to blame the physician for this; in a sense, he is a victim of the system, of insurance contracts oriented to hospital care, of the public preceptions that hospital care is the only safe care, of malpractice suits, etc.

Irving J. Lewis, in an article in *Scientific American*, puts it this way:

"The physician is motivated, by education and a kind of technological imperative, to utilize the latest procedures, the most sophisticated tests and so on. This attitude influences his decision as to who does and who does not require hospitalization, the highest-cost component of medical care. To the physician, cost considerations – the patient's or the insurance company's or the government's – are secondary to what he considers to be the best and most advanced medical practice."

If anything seems clear to me in all the debate it is that, in one way or another, the physician will once again have to exercise accountability not only with regard to quality of service but its cost. Consider it this way: the individual physician, on the average, orders up for his patients services totalling something like $250,000 each year. He is at the point of control of that flow of money. He must assume responsibility in this area or the government will do it for him. To me, it is as simple as that.

A recently released study by HEW of the Federal Employees Health Benefits program, a nation-wide program which Aetna participates in as administrator of the government-wide indemnity benefit option, shows the following 1968 utilization data: for Blue Cross-Blue Shield plans, 924 hospital days per 1,000 covered persons; for the Indemnity Plan, 987 days; for seven different prepaid group practices, 422 days. The data further show that this gap between fee-for-service and capitation payment widened between the early 1960's and 1968 – the number of days increased for the fee-for-service plans and decreased for the capitation plans.

The medical profession, despite such data, still tries to assert that the case has not been proved for prepaid group practices. To one who knows that the Kaiser doctors don't get all of their substantial year-end bonus unless they limit hospital utilization to 525 days or less of hospital care per 1,000 subscribers per year as well as keeping a lid on ancillary services, that is nonsense. If something like that same kind of financial discipline cannot be assumed by physicians who operate on fee-for-service, then, in my opinion, such physicians deserve to be put on a government salary.

I have dwelt at length on this matter of costs under the fee-for-service system because, as I'm sure you now realize, I believe firmly that our survival as health insurers depends totally on whether costs can be brought into line under the fee-for-service system. We can help in that regard, but we cannot determine the outcome. That's up to the medical profession.

The Health Insurance Association of America is supporting a National Health Insurance plan which has been introduced in the Senate by Senator McIntyre of New Hampshire and others, and in the House by Representative Burleson of Texas and others. Today, I wish to give you just the essential concepts of the bill on the theory that the less said, the more you may remember.

First, we propose several improvements relating to the organization and delivery of health care services. We recommend:

(a) That health manpower be increased in a variety of ways, particularly by increasing federal loans to students and permitting repayment of such loans by service in areas of special need;

(b) That lower-cost ambulatory care services be promoted through federal grants for the development of comprehensive ambulatory care centers;

(c) That financial support for comprehensive health planning agencies be increased and greater power given to them to combat wasteful duplication of services;

(d) That each state be required to establish by legislation public-utility-like regulation of hospitals and other health care institutions so that we can get a handle on spiralling costs; and

(e) That a Council of Health Policy Advisors analogous to the Council of Economic Advisors be created to advise the President on health matters and to articulate national goals.

With regard to financing, the HIAA plan calls for the establishment of Federal standards for health insurance companies and tax incentives for individuals and employers to meet those standards on a voluntary basis. In addition, we introduce the concept of state health insurance pools, underwritten by all insurers doing business in a state, which would provide policies meeting the federal standards to the poor, the near-poor and those with resources who cannot buy health insurance at reasonable cost because of health impairments. These state plans or pools would eventually replace Medicaid and would be funded principally as Medicaid is now, but with increased federal sharing and uniform benefits among the states. The idea is that we could get away from the welfare orientation of Medicaid if those covered by the state pool could receive private health insurance policies.

The HIAA plan would not disturb the Medicare program.

In order to offer policies meeting federal standards, all health insurers would include ambulatory care benefits in their contracts. One of the most valid criticisms of health insurers has been that they pay for certain diagnostic tests only if performed in the hospital. The problem has not been that we've been unwilling to sell such coverage but rather that our customers generally prefer to use available dollars to improve hospital coverage.

The federal benefit standards included in the HIAA bill are designed to phase in benefits during the 1970's as the services available increase to meet increased demand. In its ultimate phase, the benefit standards call for no limits on ambulatory care and very high limits on insitutional care. Benefits would cover catastrophic illnesses of almost every conceivable variety.

The HIAA plan represents a workable, pragmatic approach to the nation's health care crisis. Its chief advantage is that it could become operative almost overnight. We think some of its features are sure to be included in whatever plan ultimately emerges from Congress.

The New York Times this week had a front page story entitled, "Americans Now Favor A National Health Plan." The first paragraph reads, "Subtly but unmistakably, Americans from all strata of society and all economic classes are swinging over to the idea that good health care, like a good education, ought to be a fundamental right of citizenship."

And so, the $64 question is not whether we will have national health insurance, but *when*. And, for health insurers especially, what kind. We're confident our services will be needed, in the last analysis.

Group Practice: A Challenge to Podiatry

Donald C. Helms

In today's economic climate, operating our respective practices and organizations economically and with financial restraint is certainly a challenge and often a nightmare. It is obvious that with many of our present systems, offices may be administratively top-heavy with a large amount of available funds going to the employment of administrative personnel, secretaries and equipment, etc. Recognizing that some of these arrangements are indispensable, we plead for better direction of our financial resources toward improving our professional effectiveness in meeting the foot health needs of the community.

Group medical practice, specifically the multi-service group – is a principal avenue whereby health care may be better organized to meet the overwhelming needs of the community. The demand of the individual community, coupled with the desires and attitudes of the specialists, may create a broad range of organizational patterns. It is important to recognize that a well-trained physician or podiatrist, motivated to pursue the purpose of the group, is a prerequisite to superior group practice.

Opportunities for developing the professional capabilities of the physician and/or podiatrist are vital to the stability of the organization. These opportunities embrace the sharing of patients as well as sharing professional knowledge – and permit continuing education.

The satisfaction of a podiatrist or any practitioner within a group is dependent on many factors. Significant professional advantages are:

(1) Broad scope of consultation with other health professionals and easy accessibility.
(2) Formal and informal participation in education programs.
(3) Proper atmosphere, both physical and mental, for high quality practice and peer review.
(4) Opportunities for economical use of health manpower, resources, and facilities.

Donald C. Helms, D.P.M., *Chief, Podiatric Section, Hitchcock Clinic, Dartmouth-Hitchcock Medical Center, Hanover, New Hampshire.*

(5) Ease of managing medical problems of the total patient.

(6) Satisfactory income.

(7) Various benefit programs that produce financial security are available.

(8) Most of all it frees the podiatrist to concentrate his professional efforts on the practice he knows best, capturing more time for normal living and for study — to keep pace with his changing profession.

Podiatry, in a group setting, may be incorporated in Departments of Medicine where its specialized methods best serve the wide range of referring sources. Special relationships develop in a natural manner to include the diabetologist, rheumatologist, vascular surgeon, general surgeon, neurosurgeon, dermatologist, orthopedist, and pediatrician. In this atmosphere, in addition to the primary function of keeping normal feet in good condition, protecting high risk feet from injury and detecting and treating foot abnormalities, the podiatrist easily becomes involved in a teaching capacity for staff; in developing foot care protocols for nursing staff; training visiting nurses in home care; and instructing patients in the specialty clinics.

Meetings and discussion groups such as this are meant to encourage an evaluation of what is being done in the health care system today and what is needed in the future. Innovative proposals to meet community needs such as increasing health insurance, regional comprehensive health planning, group practice and prepaid medical plans are increasing the services available to larger numbers of people. The podiatry professional is charged with meeting his responsibility in this planning. He must evaluate his existing service wherever he is, with a view to creating a better delivery system; that is, a system which will make his programs and service more available to the people. The inclusion of various health specialists in a comprehensive system is gradually evolving across the nation. We and other professionals should be alert to making ourselves available for roles we may be asked to assume in the future. At the very least, we should cooperate in devising ways and means for superior podiatric care beyond what is now available.

III. Practical Application of Assessment Factors and Criteria for Surgical Approach to Hallux Abducto Valgus

The Surgical Treatment of Hallux Abducto Valgus

Stephen D. Smith

There have been at least 1,000 articles written on the subject of hallux abducto valgus and over 100 different types of surgical corrections and modifications for its treatment. In itself, this is testimony that there is not one, two, or three surgical procedures that are best suited for all bunion deformities.

I believe that podiatrists should concern themselves more with the etiologies creating the bunion deformity, the pathomechanics, and in understanding the progression of events that occur in the development of a hallux abducto valgus. We should also better learn to prognosticate which bunions are going to get worse, particularly when we are treating children and adolescents.

This morning we are offering a review of the literature, statistically correlated information, the application of biomechanical laws, practical experience, and some personal observations and thoughts. We are not offering by any means the complete answer to the problem of hallux abducto valgus but rather a foundation on which we can build a more sophisticated approach to the problem.

Any surgeon who is concerning himself with this problem must have a complete understanding of the different etiologies, the pathomechanics, and the procedures which are the best to correct the deformity in the particular stage that it exists and which will give the best results from the standpoint of function and cosmetics.

The underlying etiology of almost any bunion deformity is hypermobility of the first ray. Hypermobility is defined as movement occurring in a joint at a time when that joint should be stable under the load. For instance, during the propulsive phase of gait, the first metatarsal should not move in response to gravitational forces and the body weight passing through it, but if the first ray moves abnormally during the propulsion phase of gait then we get a buckling created at the metatarsal phalangeal joint and the first stages of hallux abducto valgus are set into motion.

Stephen D. Smith, D.P.M., *Clinical Instructor, Illinois College of Podiatric Medicine, Chicago, Illinois.*

Every podiatrist should be completely aware of the function of the foot, its normal variations, the deviations from normal, and, when we are concerning ourselves with hallux abducto valgus, the etiologies of the problem. The foot basically has two functions:

It serves as a pronated mobile adapter during the first part of stance phase of gait, adapting to the level of the ground, positioning the foot in such a manner that the entire plantar surface of the foot can make contact with ground, adjusting for any variances in the ground and for any deviations of the body above, accommodating for internal leg rotation and serving to absorb kinetic energy at heel contact. The foot during the first 25% of stance phase of gait is like a loose bag of bones plopping to the ground and assuming the level of the ground and the other things we have just mentioned. During the midstance phase of gait, the foot is moving from a position of being a pronated mobile adapter to a position of being a supinated rigid lever for propulsion, so that when heel off occurs and the weight is transferred to the forepart of the foot, the osseous segments are stable and capable of transmitting weight across the osseous segments. The majority of problems we see in podiatry come about because of the inability of the foot to become a rigid lever during the propulsive phase of gait. When heel off occurs, the foot is not sufficiently stable to transmit weight across the osseous elements and, therefore, through the active forces of gravity the osseous segments are moved abnormally creating shear of the metatarsals and development of hyperkeratotic lesions on the plantar surface of the foot, producing instability of the metatarsal phalangeal joint articulation with hammer toe deformity, and eventually a clavus formation. This has a particularly strong effect on the first ray, creating hypermobility of the first ray where the first ray moves abnormally and sets up a buckling force at the first metatarsal phalangeal joint articulation, initiating the first stages in the development of a hallux abducto valgus deformity. Hypermobility of the forefoot, in the majority of cases and in particular the first ray, is created by subtalar joint pronation.

We can see in the closed kinetic chain that the talus abducts and planiflexes and the calcaneus everts in the case of pronation. In supination the talus is abducted and dorsiflexed and the calcaneus is everted. Thus, we have a normal pronatory supinatory movement occurring at the subtalar joint. Subtalar joint movement controls the locking and unlocking of the midtarsal joint; this unlocking and locking of the midtarsal joint renders the forefoot either stable or hypermobile.

Midtarsal Joint Locking Mechanism

When the subtalar joint is in its neutral position, the midtarsal joint is maximally pronated and the level between 1 and 5 is parallel to the weight-bearing surface; at that time it is also perpendicular to the posterior bisection of the calcaneus. With applied force to the lateral side of the forefoot in the pronatory direction, no further pronation is available at the midtarsal joint because the subtalar joint is then in the neutral position and the midtarsal joint is locked and capable of transmitting weight across it without having osseous segments move abnormally. If a force is applied to the medial side of the forefoot, we can dorsiflex and invert the medial side of the forefoot unrestricted. There is a full range of supination at the midtarsal joint only with pressure on the medial side of the forefoot. When the subtalar joint is pronated, force can be applied to the lateral side of the forefoot in the pronatory direction, and when the midtarsal joint is maximally pronated the level between 1 and 5 is everted to the ground. We have unlocked the midtarsal joint, allowing an "extra range" of pronation so that when the midtarsal joint is maximally pronated the forefoot is everted in relation to the rear foot and to the ground. This is an unreal situation since the foot cannot transmit weight and cannot be stood on in this manner. In order to bring the lateral side of the forefoot to the ground the medial side of the forefoot is pushed out of the way. This also leaves the midtarsal joint extremely hypermobile with particular emphasis on the first ray. The underlying etiology of hallux abducto valgus deformity is usually pronation of the subtalar joint and is usually associated with locking of the midtarsal joint with hypermobility, especially of the first ray.

The first ray functions around its own axis of motion. The axis of motion of the first ray runs approximately through the tuberosity of the navicular and out through the third cuneiform. Looking at an anterior/posterior view, we see that it runs from posterior, medial, and dorsal, to anterior, lateral, and plantar. The motion that occurs around the first metatarsal is dorsiflexion, inversion, planiflexion, and eversion. There is a slight amount of abduction when the metatarsal is moved above the transverse plane. There is a small amount of adduction when the metatarsals move from the neutral position in the planiflexary direction. For practical purposes, the normal range of motion is dorsiflexion and inversion, planiflexion and eversion.

The peroneus longus muscle provides stability of the first ray on the medial side of the foot. When the subtalar joint is in the neutral position, the midtarsal joint is also in its neutral position and it is maximally pronated with the level between the first and fifth metatarsals parallel to the ground. Osseous stability exists and weight is capable of being transmitted across the midtarsal joint into the forefoot. The peroneus longus muscle can also be seen as it goes from its origin to its insertion, and as it is reflected around the body of the cuboid it goes slightly anterior, dorsal, and medial. There are, therefore, three vectors of force. It pulls back in the first ray (the first cuneiform is in the first metatarsal's), stabilizing the first ray against the tarsal area, pulling it toward the lateral side of the foot which is stable because it is on the ground. It stabilizes the first ray on the medial side of the foot to the lateral side of the foot and it is deflected dorsally; it produces planiflexion of the first ray, stabilizing the medial side of the foot to the lateral side of the foot. In a pronated position, however, the distance between the first cuneiform and the cuboid is flattened out so that now the peroneus longus muscle is capable only of producing stability posteriorly and transversely, not in a planiflex direction. It cannot planiflex and stabilize the medial side of the foot to the ground; it has flattened out that distance. Now hypermobility of the first ray exists because of the inability of the peroneus longus muscle to stabilize the first ray. If the foot fails to become a rigid lever in the propulsive phase of gait and the midtarsal joint is unlocked at that time, then the peroneus longus muscle cannot produce stability of the first ray. The first ray then dorsiflexes and everts and that sets up the first stages in the dislocating force of the first metatarsal phalangeal joint articulation. There are no muscle attachments to the head of the first metatarsal, only ligamentous attachments. The sesamoids lie in the tendons of the short flexor halluces muscle and all the other muscles. The abductor and the adductor are inserted via the sesamoids into the base of the proximal phalanx so that the head rotates out of its normal socket. The sesamoids do not migrate into the inner space. The first head moves out of the way, the capsule and ligaments along the medial side become stretched and the capsule and ligaments on the lateral side become contracted. The toe eventually goes into valgus rotation and abduction deviation. In the initial stages of development of a hallux abducto valgus deformity, the first ray is hypermobile. It dorsiflexes and inverts, setting up the first stages in the dislocation process.

We said that the majority of problems that create hypermobility of the forefoot, particularly the first ray, are those that produce pronation of the subtalar joint; anything that produces pronation of the subtalar joint unlocks the midtarsal joint and leaves the first ray hypermobile. This could be internal leg rotation, a rear foot varus, a forefoot varus, but particularly we are concerned about equinus conditions. Equinus conditions are notoriously intractable to conservative treatment. If the heel can't be kept on the ground during the stance phase of gait, no mechanical device can control the pronation created by the equinus deformity. Most people who have equinus deformities are not the classical toe-walkers that you see; it is a quantitative thing. The equinus is defined as the inability of the foot to dorsiflex a maximum of 10 degrees when the knee is extended and the subtalar joint is in a neutral position. Most people who have an equinus deformity mask it by a complex compensatory mechanism resulting in pronation of the subtalar joint. Equinus produces the worst pronation of the foot of any of the types of foot deformity. Since a congenital gastrocnemius equinus is present since birth, it has very damaging effects on the foot and can produce a juvenile hallux abducto valgus deformity. The equinus state, when it compensates, results in a severe pronation of the subtalar joint when motion is available to that joint, and the forefoot supinates on the rear foot and severe hypermobility of the first ray occurs.

There is another major force which creates dislocation of the first metatarsal phalangeal joint articulation but does not necessarily produce pronation of the subtalar joint — i.e., the forefoot valgus. When the subtalar joint is in the neutral position and the midtarsal joint is maximally pronated, the level between 1 and 5 is everted to the rear foot, and that is designated a forefoot valgus. When the forefoot valgus compensates for supination from the midtarsal joint, it leaves the fore part of the foot unlocked at the midtarsal joint and this particularly produces dysplasia and hypermobility of the first metatarsal.

Whenever you see a juvenile hallux abducto valgus, a bunion deformity in a child, look for: (1) a forefoot valgus deformity and (2) an equinus deformity. These are the two major dislocating factors in the development of bunions in children.

Another etiological agent is forefoot adductus. In the forefoot rectus type of foot, the longitudinal axis of the second metatarsal parallels the longitudinal axis of the rear foot. On x-ray we construct the longitudinal axis of the rear foot by bisecting the heel and also placing another dot at the anterior medial aspect of the calcaneus. The two dots are connected and the line is extended out through the end of the foot. Then we construct a lesser tarsus perpendicular; we place a dot at the posterior medial aspect of the first metatarsal and another dot at the anterior medial aspect of the talus where the articulating portion of bone ends or meets with the navicular. We place another dot at the posterior lateral aspect of the fourth metatarsal and at the anterior lateral aspect of the calcaneus. We bisect both lines and construct a lesser tarsus transection. Anywhere along that line, we construct a perpendicular and this gives the direction of the tarsus area. Then we bisect the longitudinal axis of the second metatarsal and also bisect the longitudinal axis of the proximal phalanx.

In the forefoot adductus type of foot, there is an exaggeration of the metatarsus adductus. The lesser tarsus perpendicular may form a normal angle with the longitudinal axis of the rear foot but there is an exaggeration of the metatarsus adductus angle which is the axis measured between the second metatarsal and the lesser tarsus perpendicular, If the angle is more than 22 degrees, it becomes pathological and a major contributing factor in the development of a hallux abducto valgus. This is because, in the rectus type of foot, all the intrinsic muscles that attach into the base of the proximal phalanx have a fairly straight course and are inserted into the base of this phalanx, approximately perpendicularly to the axis of motion of the first metatarsal phalangeal joint articulation. However, with the metatarsus adductus type of foot the angulation of the intrinsic muscles that attach into the base of the proximal phalanx are more oblique to the axis of rotation of the first metatarsal phalangeal joint; therefore, this produces an adduction deviation to the proximal phalanx. The adductor muscle pulls to the base of the proximal phalanx laterally; the abductor muscle slides underneath the condyle. Instead of producing stability in the transverse plane, it now produces planiflexion of the medial side of the proximal phalanx which creates valgus rotation. The short flexor tendons are now more lateral to the axis of motion in the first metatarsal phalangeal joint articulation. The lateral head of the short flexor containing a lateral sesamoid is now producing abduction deviation to the proximal phalanx; the medial head of the short flexor tendon is also producing planiflexion on the medial aspect of the proximal phalanx increasing valgus deviation of the toe. A sesamoid which is located in the lateral head of the short flexor is also acting as a fulcrum to increase the abductor force of the lateral head of that muscle. The long and short flexors are not running underneath and parallel to the bone directly underneath the axis of motion but are now bowstrung across the joint increasing the abduction deviation of the hallux.

In the initial stages of hallux abducto valgus there is abduction deviation; when the hallux abductus angle gets to be about 30 degrees, valgus rotation begins.

The range of motion of the first metatarsal phalangeal joint is dependent upon the range of motion of the first ray. If the first ray is to be stabilized in its neutral position, that is, halfway along its range of motion and then move the metatarsal phalangeal joint, there would be about 45 degrees of dorsiflexion and 25 degrees of planiflexion. However, that does not happen during gait. During the first portion of the stance phase of gait the first metatarsal is elevated and, therefore, there is limitation of dorsiflexion at the metatarsal phalangeal joint and an increased range of planiflexion. As the first metatarsal is planiflexed during the propulsive portion of the stance phase of gait, the first metatarsal becomes planiflexed and, therefore, planiflexion is limited and dorsiflexion increased. This is one of the major causes of limitation and development of hallux rigidus. I have never seen a hallux rigidus that did not have an elevatus of the first ray. By producing an elevatus of the first ray, the dorsiflexion range of motion is decreased and jamming of the dorsal aspect of the joint occurs with eventual osteophytic proliferation and hallux rigidus deformity.

The range of motion of the first metatarsal is dependent on the plantar fascia. In a normal foot in its neutral position, there is some slack in the plantar fascia when the toe is extended off the metatarsal. However, if the proximal phalanx were dorsiflexed in relation to the first metatarsal, the slack in the tendon would be taken up and there would be tension produced by the plantar fascia limiting dorsiflexion of the proximal phalanx. Also, as soon as the heel leaves the ground there is produced a supinatory effect on the subtalar joint since the plantar fascia is attached into the digit, so the purpose of the plantar fascia is to prevent dislocation of the digits during the propulsive phase of gait and to aid in supination of the subtalar joint after heel off, and not to support the longitudinal metatarsal arch.

When there is a pes cavus type of foot, or a supinated foot, there is an increased pitch of the first metatarsal, an increased range of dorsiflexion of the proximal phalanx. When the foot is supinated the distance between the first metatarsal head and the calcaneal tuberosity is lessened, which puts more slack in the tendon and allows for more dorsiflexion in the toe to occur. One of the major causes of hallux abducto valgus is pronation of the subtalar joint and with the pronation of that joint there is elevatus of the first metatarsal. So, in the propulsive phase of gait, the first metatarsal is dorsiflexed and inverted instead of being plantar flexed. This decreases the distance between the origin and insertion of the plantar fascia so that when the heel lifts off the ground, plantar flexion of the first metatarsal does not occur. Therefore, there is a limitation of dorsiflexion and the proximal phalanx is jammed into the dorsal aspect of the metatarsal and osteophytic proliferation occurs.

Another contributing factor to the development of hallux abducto valgus is the type of first metatarsal head that is involved. The head of the first metatarsal is either round square, or square with a center ridge. The worst set of circumstances I can think of to predispose someone to hallux abducto valgus deformity is an equinus deformity with a non-rigid forefoot valgus, a metatarsus adductus, and a round first metatarsal head. It is easier for the base of the proximal phalanx to slip off the head of the first metatarsal when the head is round; it is harder for the first metatarsal to dislocate when there is a square first metatarsal head.

A head of the first metatarsal with a center ridge is the best type to have because even with moderate hypermobility of the first ray, dislocation will be less likely because it is difficult to dislocate the proximal phalanx on the head of the metatarsal when there is a center groove.

When we examine a bunion, we should ask ourselves: what is the cause of the bunion; what force produced the hypermobility of the first metatarsal of the first ray and began the dislocation process; what stage of development is the condition in; will it tend to get worse? From the radiographs we want to determine if the deviation position, or buckling, of the joint is structural or positional in nature? What I mean by positional is that there is a dynamic muscle imbalance. All the deformity is occurring at the joint itself! There is an alteration in the relationship of the proximal phalanx to the first metatarsal head. The structural nature of the deformity will be discussed later.

Joints are classified into three types: (1) congruous; (2) deviated; and (3) sublux. In a congruous joint, the joint surfaces are parallel and even and the center of the base of the proximal phalanx opposes the center of the first metatarsal head. In the deviated type of joint, when lines are constructed representing the two joint surfaces, they form an angle outside the joint. The sublux type of joint can be identified by constructing lines representing the articulating portion of bone at the base of the proximal phalanx and at the head of the first metatarsal. When the lines cross and form an angle inside the joint, the joint is a subluxed type of joint.

The normal range of a deviated joint is from 15-35 degrees. The H.A. (hallux abductus) Angle is found by bisecting the proximal phalanx and constructing the longitudinal axis of the first metatarsal. Where these bisections cross, this is known as the H.A. Angle. The H.A. Angle is normally 10-15 degrees when the joint surfaces are congruous. Why should there be an H.A. Angle of 10-15 degrees when you would expect the articulating surface of any long bone to be perpendicular to the long axis of its supporting bone? In the case of the first metatarsal phalangeal joint, the first metatarsal, and the proximal phalanx, the articulating portion of bone at the head of the metatarsal is slightly oblique to the long axis of the supporting bone. Also, the shaft of the proximal phalanx is angulated. This is why there is a normal H.A. Angle of 10-15 degrees with the joint surfaces being congruous. There is an oblique setting of the articulating portion of bone at the head of the first metatarsal and a deviation of the proximal phalanx relation to its articulating portion of bone.

In the first stages of a bunion deformity, there is dorsiflexion and inversion of the first metatarsal. Since the base of the proximal phalanx cannot be stabilized on the head of the first metatarsal, there is slight lateral and plantar movement. Bone has greater resistance to compression than it has to stress. When there is increased stress within physiological limits on the lateral side, bone growth is stimulated and the ligaments are stretched. When there is stress beyond its resistence, then erosion of bone takes place. The sagittal groove is formed by either the gouging in of the base of the proximal phalanx or by disuse atrophy where there has been no pressure, but eventually there is remodeling of the articular facet. It is possible to have a completely congruous joint with an increase in the H.A. Angle leaving the medial head of the first metatarsal exposed to shoe trauma, especially if there is hypermobility present. Therefore, you can have all of the symptoms of a bunion with a completely congruous joint.

In one case the epiphyses have not quite closed and there is functional bone adaptation where the articulating portion of the bone at the head of the first metatarsal is more than 5-8 degrees, but there is a fairly congruous joint. If a soft tissue correction were done to straighten the proximal phalanx on the metatarsal head, wedging of the joint would occur and the joint surfaces would be deviated to the other side.

Limitation of dorsiflexion does not usually occur because of soft tissue contraction; it occurs when the base of the proximal phalanx is articulating across the bias because of functional bone adaptation which has taken place at the head of the first metatarsal. When there is a bone or a joint articulating obliquely to the axis of motion, there is limitation of motion. Also, if nothing is done to alleviate elevatus or dorsiflexion of the ray, plantar fascia also limits dorsiflexion.

The I.M. (Inter Metatarsal) Angle represents the amount of deviation of the first metatarsal from the second metatarsal. It is constructed by bisecting the longitudinal axis of the second metatarsal and bisecting the longitudinal axis of the first metatarsal; where the lines meet and form an angle is called the I.M. angle. The normal is about 7.1.

In small hallux valgus deformities, there is about a 2:1 relationship of the inter metatarsal angle with the H. A. Angle. The normal H.A. Angle is 15 degrees and the normal I.M. Angle is 7 degrees. This is a 2:1 relationship; if there is a 10 degree I.M. Angle you may expect a 20 degree H.A. Angle. When the angles are greater this relationship does not hold because once the subluxation process is set into motion, it is difficult to stop and the H.A. Angle may easily reach 50-60 degrees. The H.A. Angle, when the joint surfaces are parallel and congruous, should equal the addition of the proximal articular set angle and the distal articular set angle.

The entire increase in the normal angle is due to deviation at the joint itself. In almost any bunion deformity, you can add up the joint angle, the proximal and distal articular set angles to equal the H.A. Angle.

The entire 20 degree deviation is due to subluxation of the joint. The joint surfaces form an angle inside the joint so it is a sublux joint.

So these are three different kinds of bunion deformities. All with the same H.A. Angle but with different elements; one is all structural, one is structural and positional, one is all positional. It makes a difference in the kind of correction that should be used. When we straighten a toe when the joint is congruous and the whole deviation is structural in nature, there is an increase in the proximal articular set angles, we will have wedging at the joint and the joint will be deviated to the other side. The H.A. Angle is normally 5-20 degrees; from 20-30 degrees is a mild deviation.

When we are dealing with a congruous type of joint, the H.A. Angle is usually from 5-25 degrees, mode of 15 degrees; the intermetatarsal angle is about 8 degrees; there is no deviation of the sesamoids; there is no valgus rotation. In a deviated type of joint, the H.A. is about 13-35 degrees, mode of about 25 degrees; an I.M. Angle of 5-7 degrees, mode of about 11 degrees. In the sublux type of joint, the H.A. Angle is from 20-60 degrees; intermetatarsal angle of 8-20 degrees; mode of about 14 degrees.

A congruous type of joint with a bunion deformity does not represent an earlier stage of the other two types but a deviated type of joint is an earlier stage of the sublux type. For example, a female, age 13, who has a mild equinus, hypermobility of the first ray, a round first metatarsal head and a little metatarsus adductus and a deviated joint will, by the time she is 35, have a sublux joint. The joint is better treated early. However, when another female is seen with a congruous type of joint; the likelihood of its worsening is not great.

Likewise, a deviated joint in an adult 40 years old would not be expected to worsen but a subluxed joint at any age is always progressive.

Another subject with which we are concerned is relative metatarsal protrusion, that is, the relative length of the first metatarsal to the second metatarsal. Normally, the first and second metatarsals are equal in length within 1 or 2 millimeters. Metatarsal protrusion is measured by bisecting the longitudinal axis of the second metatarsal and the first metatarsal where they come together at an apex. You place the pointed end of a compass, then you stretch out the pencil to the length of the first metatarsal and construct a small arc over the second. Then you stretch out the compass to the second metatarsal head and construct a small arc.

In one case, the first metatarsal is longer than the second metatarsal. What is the importance of the relative metatarsal protrusion? It is important in deciding on an operative procedure. In one case, we would like to take away length of the first metatarsal; it helps us to determine whether we are going to do an opening or closing abductory osteotomy of the first metatarsal and what kind of a drain orthoplasia should be done — Keller, Stone, or Mayo.

In another case, the first and second metatarsals are of equal length. Several degrees of reduction in the I.M. Angle can be expected by just a soft tissue correction. If the first metatarsal is going to reduce in its I.M. Angle, then the relative metatarsal protrusion is going to effect a change at the metatarsal phalangeal joint. Hardy Clapman found that when there is a long first metatarsal, there is a tendency for a low I.M. Angle and a large H.A. Angle and that is usually associated with the round type joint and a mild metatarsus adductus. When there is a short first metatarsal, there is usually a larger I.M. Angle and a smaller H.A. Angle than is expected. What is the importance of this? Let us consider a 20-year-old female patient with a deviated joint. An arthroplasty would not be considered. The I.M. Angle would not be large enough for an osteotomy but we know it is going to get worse — we would prefer to do a soft tissue correction. What things are likely to happen if hypermobility exists and it can't be controlled? If the first metatarsal head is longer, then we should do an adductory release. When the first metatarsal head is long it gives an additional fulcrum to the hallux and the second toe is not an effective buttress to the buckling of the first metatarsal phalangeal joint, so there is a tendency for larger H.A. Angles and smaller I.M. Angles. When the first metatarsal is shorter, the second toe is an effective buttress to the lateral deviation of the hallux so that a retrograde force is produced in the first metatarsal and produces an increase in the I.M. Angle. If you are going to do a soft tissue correction of the short first metatarsal, it is well to transfer the abductors to the head of the first metatarsal to help move it and reduce the I.M. Angle. This is not necessary if you have a long first metatarsal because you won't get a large I.M. Angle; we usually do two lengthenings on the adductors.

Interphalangus

Interphalangus can be produced by asymmetry of the distal phalanx where the medial cortex is longer than the lateral cortex so that the toe deviates in the distal phalanx. There can also be an oblique setting of the head of the proximal phalanx so that there is tilting of the portion of bone at the head of the proximal phalanx in relation to the long axis of the supporting bone. There can be lateral tilting of the articulating surface of bone which pushes the distal phalanx lateralward. It is better to do an osteotomy which is fairly atraumatic, does not disrupt function and straightens the interphalangus than to do a soft tissue correction which may result in overcorrection and deviation of the metatarsal phalangeal joint without taking into account the interphalangus.

Adduction Deviation

This is asymmetry of the distal phalanx where the articulating portion of bone at the head of the proximal phalanx is perpendicular to the long axis of the supporting bone but the cortex is longer on the medial side than the lateral side which produces an interphalangus appearance. The hallux appears to be in abduction but actually the joints are parallel and congruous.

The Sesamoid's Position

In the past, the rule of thumb was that you removed the lateral sesamoid when it was more than half displaced. It is difficult to be sure where the lateral sesamoid is in relation to the metatarsal because it is usually moving in a sagittal direction so that it is parallel to the center of the x-ray beam. The tibial sesamoid, on the other hand, is always on the frontal plane, a transverse plane, and perpendicular to the center of the x-ray. It is in a thick fibrous cartilaginous ligament binding the two sesamoids together, called the intersesamoid ligament. The fibular sesamoid isn't going to be going anywhere. The tibial sesamoid isn't going.

Summary

Some of the criteria and assessment factors in the evaluation of patients with hallux abducto valgus deformity have been presented. We should look at bunions from the viewpoint of their etiology, the force creating the buckling of the first metatarsal phalangeal joint articulation, the stage of development presenting, the prognosis if the bunion is untreated. By assessing these factors, we can better determine what type of operation should be performed on that joint to give the most desirable functional and cosmetic end result.

The Surgical Correction of Hallux Abducto Valgus

Lowell Scott Weil

Most of the criteria we will mention have been developed through our experience and study and are the result of attempts to adhere to the principles of biomechanics and avoidance of repetition of errors. We also believe that the patient should be assessed as an individual, and not as a statistic or as an x-ray picture. The proper procedure must be applied to the individual patient.

Dr. Smith has reviewed some of the criteria used in assessment of a particular case. These included: (1) the sex of the patient and the type of footwear the patient would want to wear postoperatively; (2) age – some procedures might be better for the elderly than the younger patient; (3) occupation; (4) general level of activity of the patient; (5) the etiological force, such as equinus or nonrigid forefoot valgus; a severe force on the first metatarsal has to be dealt with differently than other types of forces.

There are other specific considerations which have to be taken into account, and which were mentioned by Dr. Smith:

(1) The presence or absence of an arthritic joint. An arthritic joint is now cared for by some type of arthroplasty such as a Stone, modified Mayo, or modified Keller procedure. When there is an arthritic joint, it is very difficult to maintain any type of congruity between the joint surfaces or to obtain a good range of motion postoperatively. One can get a straight joint but it may not work very well.

(2) Articular set angle

(3) Digital length pattern – we may wish to shorten a particular segment

(4) The forefoot type, whether it is an adductus or rectus foot.

(5) Hallux abductus angle

(6) Hallux abductus interphalangeal angle

(7) Intermetatarsal angle

(8) Joint congruity

Lowell Scott Weil, D.P.M., *Instructor in Biomechanics, Illinois College of Podiatric Medicine, Chicago, Ill.*

(9) Long axis of the rear foot — in the normal foot the long axis of the digits should parallel the long axis of the rear foot. Whenever we attempt to correct a hallux abducto valgus deformity, this orientation should be kept in mind. The hallux will always attempt to simulate this position paralleling the long axis of the rear foot. This principle comes into play particularly when treating a metatarsus adductus condition, either mild or moderate, or forefoot adductus condition. Too often we try to place the hallux in a position which appears straight with the first metatarsal rather than parallel with the long axis of the rear foot.

(10) Relative metatarsus adductus angle

(11) Relative metatarsus protrusion

(12) The range and direction of motion of the first metatarsal phalangeal joint

(13) Relative forefoot adductus

(14) The shape of the crista. We have found that wearing away of the crista allows for very quick deviation of the hallux and it is difficult to reposition the medial and lateral sesamoids when the crista has been completely eroded; they tend to go back into a deviated position.

(15) Shape of the first metatarsal head

(16) The tibial sesamoid position.

We have divided our surgical procedures into five categories: (1) simple exostectomy; (2) simple exostectomy with soft tissue correction; (3) arthroplasty; (4) osteotomy; (5) arthrodesis.

We feel that the simple exostectomy, the Silver procedure, should be used almost exclusively in the elderly, debilitated patient with a very severe deformity, especially when it is complicated by another chronic condition such as a sinus. The procedure is used only to relieve symptoms. The condition of a 70-year-old patient with a very prominent medial aspect of the first metatarsal head was complicated by a constantly infected, very painful chronic sinus. Palliation measures failed to correct the condition so a simple exostectomy was carried out without any attempt to correct any other part of the joint. Relief of pressure was all that was necessary in this case.

The simple exostectomy with soft tissue correction is used in some selected patients. It is similar to the Silver procedure with an adductor release. We try to confine its use to younger patients between 25-40 years of age who have an intermetatarsal angle of less than $12°$ in a rectus type of foot, or an intermetatarsal angle of $10°$ or less in an adductus type of foot. The hallux abductus angle must be less than $30°$, the tibial sesamoid position must be less than $4°$ and the patient should have a square or ridge type of joint as opposed to a rounded joint. This is a very good procedure on a moderate metatarsus adductus where you just have a prominent medial aspect. In this type of case we'll do a simple exostectomy and also release the adductor structures, either through the joint or through a separate incision.

In the hope of holding a postoperative sesamoid position of about 3 in a very young patient, we did a capsulorrhaphy in this particular procedure, shortening the capsule on the medial aspect of the joint. This is necessary to change the deviated type joint. When it is a congruous joint, we would not wish to change the position of the proximal base on the head of the first metatarsal.

The most popular procedure in the podiatry profession today is the McBride procedure. This is used in persons from age 18 to 55 years of age, and we would like to have a range of motion of at least 45 degrees of dorsiflexion before we would consider this procedure. One of our observations is that a better range of motion is obtained postoperatively when the sesamoids are not removed. The tibial sesamoid position should be 4 or more; the intermetatarsal angle should be less than 14; the hallux abductus angle should be 20-35 degrees. In our experience the intermetatarsal angle has been reduced by 2 to 3 degrees in a forefoot varus type of foot and 4 to 5 degrees in a forefoot valgus type of foot with the McBride procedure.

Postoperatively, removal of the sesamoid corrected the deviation of the joint. Actually, in this case, there was slight wedging present. We refer to wedging as the point at the medial distal aspect of the first metatarsal reaching the base of the medial aspect of the base of the proximal phalanx. When we have this bone on bone contact, we refer to it as wedging, or jamming of the joint. This will limit dorsiflexion, as is seen so often after the McBride procedure. In most cases, probably another procedure should have been carried out. However, with good technical skills and good technicians, the McBride procedure can probably help solve many hallux abducto valgus problems. You can probably hold the base of the proximal phalanx in alignment with the first metatarsal and offset almost any force coming in but the technical aspect is very limited since there is often limitation of motion due to a jammed joint. This is the greatest disadvantage of the McBride procedure. The toes are nice and straight but they do not participate very much in the active phases of gait.

In one case where we performed the McBride procedure, the Akin procedure should have been done. There is a structural deformity in the base of the proximal phalanx. The surgeon placed the hallux in a straight position in relation to the first metatarsal and, of course, overcorrected it with deviation in a varus or adductus position.

When performing an exostectomy on the medial aspect of the first metatarsal, the exostosis should be removed in a dorsal medial direction rather than strictly a medial direction. Otherwise, there is no place for the medial sesamoid to articulate and it can very easily slip around to the medial side of the first metatarsal head.

In many cases of wedging of the joint following a McBride procedure, these cases culminate 2-3 years postoperatively in a hallux rigidus and end up having an orthoplasty procedure performed.

In a case of functional bony adaptation of the side of the first metatarsal head, a surgical attempt was made to correct this with a McBride procedure. The toe was straightened very well but there is no way for the toe to work very well because of the lack of an articulating surface

The Hiss procedure is another soft tissue procedure that we occasionally use. This involves a transfer of the abductor hallucis tendon. As we correct a hallux abducto valgus deformity, the tendon of the abductor hallucis begins to slide medially and plantarly under the first metatarsal head. Frequently, we find the tendon out of position. It is replaced in its proper position, and the medial aspect of the first metatarsal is reinforced.

When the abductor hallucis tendon is isolated, it is carefully dissected free from its extracapsular position. The capsular approach has been made in the usual linear direction. For our McBride procedures we prefer to use two longitudinal semi-elliptical incisions in the capsule. We remove as much tissue as necessary to correct the deviation of the joint. The higher the hallux abductus angle, the more encapsulated tissue is removed from the joint; the less the angle, the less tissue we have to remove. Exostosis is removed after the tendon has been retracted. We now reach through the joint to perform an adductor release. We do this right through the joint and cut the fibular sesamoid apparatus. The capsular structures have already been sutured and closed and the hallux is placed in proper position. It is then reinforced using the abductor tendon. We find this procedure valuable in a forefoot valgus type of foot where there is a great dislocation and hypermobility force of the first ray. A little better reinforcement is obtained by adding the abductor hallucis tendon from the side of the joint.

The Stone procedure, a partial arthroplasty of the first metatarsal head, is used in patients in the 40-60 year old age group who generally have an arthritic joint. We find this procedure best used in cases of hallux abductus limitus — where there is less than 35 degrees of dorsiflexion. The hallux abductus angle is less than 35 degrees and in its inner metatarsal angle is less than 15 degrees. In conditions with greater than 35 degrees, another arthroplasty procedure is indicated.

The modified Mayo procedure, in which there is a partial resection of the head of the first metatarsal, is used in arthritic type of joints. We remove approximately one-half of the head of the first metatarsal and remodel it to accept the base of the proximal phalanx. The inner metatarsal angle is between 12 and 17 degrees; the hallux abductus angle is 35 degrees or more. The relative metatarsal protrusion shows the first metatarsal to be longer than the second metatarsal. The modified Mayo procedure will relax the joint and allow good motion. The complications are well known: metatarsalalgia, sub-second metatarsal, inability to forcibly propel for a long period of time and, of course, the complication of osteoarthritic proliferation on the base of the proximal phalanx which could result in arthrodesis or limitus of the first metatarsal.

On an arthritic joint with a hallux abductus angle greater than 35 degrees, a partial Mayo was performed to accept the base of the proximal phalanx, removing about 2-3 millimeters of bone; the procedure worked very well.

On a partial Mayo procedure, the sesamoids were left in position and no problems are encountered.

One patient had multiple procedures performed, including the old-time Keller, with two-thirds of the base of the proximal phalanx removed in the right foot. Although we did not see the patient's x-rays preoperatively, I am certain that the first metatarsal was much longer than the second. A Keller procedure was performed. However, we were required later to do a full Mayo procedure.

Most of the criteria for a modified Keller procedure are similar to those for a Mayo procedure and the range of motion is less than 45 degrees. The modified Keller procedure is used when the relative metatarsal protrusion shows the second metatarsal to be longer than the first metatarsal and we do not wish to shorten the first metatarsal any more. We, however, do suggest some modifications in this procedure: (1) We prefer complete medial approach. There is easier access then to the base of the proximal phalanx and the structures about the base of this phalanx are very delicate and easily scarred, shredded, etc. (2) After a medial approach, any contracture we might get from a scar would only tend to pull the toe into proper position. After a dorsal approach, any contracture of the scar could pull the toe into a dorsally dislocated position. We also prefer to lengthen the extensor tendons when doing this procedure and we suture these tendons postoperatively into the capsule of the first metatarsal phalangeal joint while an assistant is holding the digit slightly plantarflexed. This is done so we are not fooled by the relaxed position of the digit, slightly dorsiflexed, on the operating table. The important result is getting the toe on the ground with plantarflexion.

Another modification of the Keller procedure is to leave the intrinsic musculature intact. This is done by performing the procedure with an oblique osteotomy of 45 degrees. The musculature is not disturbed while dissection is carried out on the medial and dorsal aspects of the base of the proximal phalanx. An oblique osteotomy is made on the base of the proximal phalanx of approximately 45 degrees. This could be referred to as a reverse Stone procedure. This allows for a great deal of dorsiflexion of the digit on to the metatarsal.

In a complete Keller procedure, the oblique osteotomy can only be utilized in cases in which the hallux abductus angle is 35-40 degrees or less. At angles greater than this, a complete Keller procedure is required. The approach is made from the medial side. When we do a complete Keller procedure, we use a Kirschner wire for 24-48 hours which is enough time to leave the gap open to fill in with hematoma, fibrous clot, etc. A shelf is left, so that the intrinsic musculature remains intact. The patient can actively propel 3-4 weeks postoperatively. The intrinsic musculature will pull the plantar aspect of the base of the proximal phalanx slightly under the head of the first metatarsal but not sufficiently to limit any type of motion.

At this point, I would like to review osteotomy procedures which include the Akin procedure, C.A.W.O. [closing abductory wedge osteotomy], O.A.W.O. [opening abductory wedge osteotomy], D.O. [double osteotomy], and D.R.A.T.O. [de rotational angulational transpositional osteotomy]. The silastic implants by Dow-Corning have been very useful in those cases in which a hallux rigidus has developed, especially those cases of postoperative McBrides that have caused a jammed joint and a fusion of the metatarsal phalangeal joint. This we have used in younger persons where a long life of mobility would be expected. Otherwise, we would have normally performed an arthroplasty such as the Mayo procedure. When we use the Akin procedure, we would have a structural deformity of the proximal phalanx of the hallux in which we would have a deviation of the distal aspect into an abductive position. A distal articular set angle of greater than 13 will usually dictate an Akin procedure performed in conjunction with some other type of soft tissue procedure. The Akin procedure is seldom performed alone. The deformity may be at the proximal phalanx, the shape of the proximal phalanx, or, as Dr. Smith mentioned, at the articulation of the interphalangeal joint.

When there is a deviation of the distal aspect of the hallux to an abductive position, an osteotomy at the base of the proximal phalanx retains the congruity of the joint and pulls the hallux into the proper position.

On removing a wedge of bone, it is rarely performed as an isolated procedure, a medial approach is made along the base of the proximal phalanx with an incision made right down to the bone, the periosteum is freed and the wedge of bone, previously determined depending on the amount of correction required, is removed leaving the lateral cortex intact. The osteotomy is closed. Two drill holes are placed, one on the distal and one on the proximal aspect into which 28 gauge monofilament wire is inserted and fixatied. The hallux is now in a relatively straight position. Congruity of the joint is maintained and a good cosmetic result will be obtained.

In another case, the Akin procedure was performed. The shape of the proximal phalanx is such that it is longer on its medial aspect and shorter on its lateral aspect. The Akin procedure maintains the congruity of the joint. Preoperatively, there was a relatively congruous joint slightly deviated. The deviation was repaired by soft tissue correction and the toe has now been placed in a proper position with the Akin procedure. If we had attempted to straighten out the toe completely by soft tissue correction, we would have had another wedged joint.

In one case with a severe deviation at the distal aspect, we performed an osteotomy a little more distally because the deviation was at the distal aspect.

The closing abductory wedge osteotomy is used in patients age 45 or younger, although the age range is quite variable. For example, in a very active 50-year-old we could consider the procedure, although it does necessitate some disability. In patients in the 50-55 year old range who are not really going to be functioning in a true gait cycle as we know it, we will often employ an arthroplasty type of procedure strictly for the convenience of the patient. Criteria are: the intermetatarsal joint angle is greater than 15 in a rectus type of foot or an inner metatarsal angle greater than 13 in an adductus type of foot. Metatarsal protrusion shows the first metatarsal to be longer. There is usually a round first metatarsal head with little to no functional bony adaptation at the lateral aspect of the first metatarsal head. We would have a deviated or mildly subluxated joint. This procedure is often used in conjunction with a McBride type of procedure. A wedge of bone is removed approximately one centimeter distal to the base of the first metatarsal and the first metatarsal is pulled into an adductory direction.

A Silver procedure was performed on a 28-year-old female with an equinus condition completely unrecognized and untouched. After the Silver procedure her bunion got worse, of course, since the medial side of the capsule was weakened. Also, the first and second metatarsal heads were tied together. We did T.A.L.'s, closing abductory wedge osteotomy, and gave her an intermetatarsal angle of 4 to 5 degrees. Actually, we got a little overzealous and we got a little wedging in the medial aspect of the joint but motion was excellent in this particular patient. We could not consider doing that procedure without first doing Achilles' tendon lengthenings. I am very reluctant to undertake bunion surgery in the face of an equinus without releasing the force of the equinus.

In subluxation of a joint resulting in surgical overcorrection, there is necessity to emphasize the need for careful calculations in performing these procedures. There are geometric and trigonometric calculations to be performed to determine exactly how much bone is to be removed and what result can be expected. In a particular patient, she was left with an intermetatarsal angle of minus 4, a hallux abductus, and a lot of problems. Of course, she was reoperated, an osteotomy performed in the other direction, and the condition was corrected.

Opening abductory osteotomy is used where there is a short first metatarsal. An attempt is made to make the first metatarsal longer as far as relative metatarsal protrusion is concerned. Usually the exostosis is used to insert into the base of the proximal phalanx after an ostoeotomy cut has been made.

In another patient who had a metatarsus adductus, all of the metatarsals were corrected in this case. Since there was a short first metatarsal, we inserted a wedge of bone in this particular area. Six months postoperatively, healing was progressing well. The first metatarsal was now in proper position by the STAMM procedure used rather than the closing abductory osteotomy which would make the bone even shorter. The STAMM is used with severe deformities, with severely subluxated joint, with arthritic processes, and a very high intermetatarsal angle. In this procedure, an arthroplasty at the metatarsal phalangeal joint is performed and the intermetatarsal angle is reduced.

In a case in which a double osteotomy has to be performed, the double osteotomy has its indications just as the closing abductory wedge osteotomy does. In another case where there was a congruous or a slightly deviated joint, the proximal articular set was 13 or greater and there was a great deal of bony adaptation on the lateral aspect of the head of the first metatarsal; if a closing abductory wedge osteotomy were performed in this case, the articular surface would be pointing even more lateralward. A double osteotomy is performed so that the articular surface would be congruous with the base of the proximal phalanx.

In the case of a young woman who wished to get back on her feet quickly, a McBride procedure was performed. Immediately postoperatively the results appeared fairly good. There was a congruous joint and there was still a slight deviation of the hallux. As time went on, however, she got worse with some rotation of the distal segment. She had to have another operation and she lost more time than if the proper procedure had been done in the first place, probably a double osteotomy. She did end up with a good functional straight toe.

The DRATO [de rotational angulational transpositional osteotomy] procedure is used on patients 40-years-old or younger with an intermetatarsal angle of less than 12 or when the range of motion is not in the sagittal plane. The joint is congruous or slightly deviated. In this procedure, a straight osteotomy is made through the entire bone. It is then rotated into an everted position. A wedge of bone is removed to adduct the articular surface and then it is slightly plantar flexed.

Arthrodesis is limited to cases of talipes in which there is a very hypermobile flexible first metatarsal. We find this condition common in many mongoloid and brain-damaged patients. We perform an arthrodesis or bunion procedure in conjunction with our closing osteotomy where we arthrodese the first metatarsal to the first cuneiform.

IV. Drug Interactions

Drug Interactions in the Podiatric Patient

Along with the recent emphasis on the use of a wider array of medications for the management of disorders of the lower extremities, there has been a growing concern about iatrogenic problems. These drug-induced difficulties often develop in a subtle fashion and are occurring with increasing frequency. The advent of new specific and potent drugs which exert their action via the alteration of certain basic cellular functions is primarily responsible for the increased evidence of drug related problems. In addition it is evident that many patients take a number of drugs simultaneously for related or unrelated disorders. These medications may include those prescribed by different medical specialists as well as certain over-the-counter drugs. The problem may be compounded in a hospital setting where the average patient receives six to ten drugs simultaneously. It has been estimated that 18% to 30% of all hospitalized patients have a drug reaction and that 3% to 5% of all admissions to hospitals are primarily for a drug reaction.

Of the undesirable drug reactions that have been reported, a growing number have involved interactions between drugs, where the effects of one drug are altered by the prior or concurrent administration of a second drug.

In order to properly consider the drug interaction problem as it applies to podiatry, it will be beneficial to briefly review the three basic types of incompatibility. The first two have long been recognized and require only brief mention here. These include "physical" incompatibilities and "chemical" incompatibilities. Podiatric examples of the former include such things as the simultaneous use of topical ointments and powders, and the mixing of oil-base and water-base products. Hence, a physical incompatibility results when there is an undesirable change in the physical state of the individual drugs or vehicles upon mixing.

Daniel A. Hussar, Ph.D., *Director of the Department of Pharmacy;*

A chemical incompatibility results when there is a chemical interaction between components of a mixture of drugs. An example would be the inactivation of quaternary ammonium type antiseptics like benzalkonium chloride (Zephiran) by soap.

Other physical and chemical incompatibilities may arise in podiatric medicine when certain topical agents are applied simultaneously to a single site or when different chemical classes of caustics and escharotics are used together (e.g., mono-, bi-, and tri-chloroacetic acid with silver nitrate or cantharidin). It should also be noted that, contrary to popular opinion, 50% alcohol or castor oil does not *chemically* neutralize topically applied phenol. These agents simply act as solvents for phenol and permit its ready dissolution so that it may easily be wiped away. Phenol skin burns can actually be spread by the use of 50% alcohol and caution must be exercised in being sure that the phenol is blotted away by gauze saturated in this solvent. Phenol is still commonly used in nail root eradication in podiatry; hence, particular note should be taken of these comments.

The third type of incompatibility is the therapeutic incompatibility. Problems relating to overdosage, adverse drug reactions and undesirable drug interactions would be included in this category. It is the purpose of this paper to review the reports of drug interactions, particularly as they apply to podiatric medicine.

Although it is often thought that all drug interactions are undesirable and represent therapeutic incompatibilities, it should be noted that sometimes a second drug is prescribed deliberately to modify the effects of another so that a beneficial interaction results. Such an approach might be utilized in an effort to enhance the effectiveness or to reduce the adverse effects of the primary agent.

Although there has been extensive publicity regarding drug interactions during the last several years, much remains to be learned. Caution is needed, therefore, in evaluating and using the information available because by misusing information or by over-reacting to a possible problem, a more difficult situation might result than what would have occurred if nothing were done.

In most cases, two drugs that are known to interact can be administered concurrently as long as adequate precautions are taken (e.g., closer monitoring of therapy, dosage adjustments to compensate for the altered response). Although there are situations where the use of one drug is usually contra-indicated while another is being given, such combinations are not likely to be employed frequently.

Therefore, drug interactions should be viewed in perspective. Although an altered response appears likely, it might not be clinically significant in many patients. In these situations, a patient should not be deprived of needed therapy because of the possibility of an interaction, but such therapy should be closely monitored.

The list of reported drug interactions has become too long to try to commit them all to memory. However, a basic understanding of the mechanisms by which these interactions develop will be valuable in anticipating such situations and in dealing with problems that do develop. Some of these mechanisms are discussed below and portrayed in Figure 1.

Drugs Having Opposing Pharmacological Effects

Interactions resulting from the use of two drugs that have opposing pharmacological effects should be among the easiest to detect. However, there may be factors that could preclude early identification of such antagonism. For example, an ophthalmologist may prescribe pilocarpine eye drops (a cholinergic agent) for a patient who is also taking an anticholinergic preparation [e.g.,

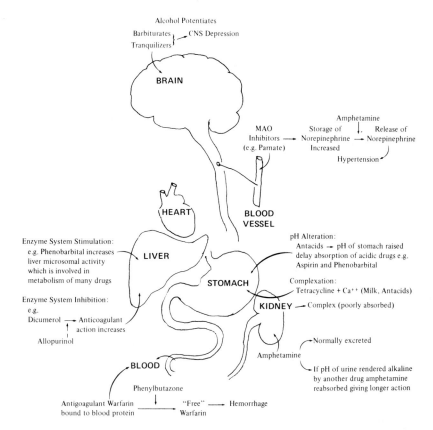

Figure 1.

propantheline (Pro-Banthine)] prescribed by another physician for a gastro-intestinal condition.

Drugs Having Similar Pharmacological Effects

This type of interaction can usually also be readily recognized. The increased central nervous system depressant effect that is experienced by individuals being treated with sedative-hypnotic drugs or tranquilizers when they consume alcoholic beverages would be an example of this type of situation.

Combined therapy with a phenothiazine tranquilizer [e.g., chlorpromazine (Thorazine)], a tricyclic antidepressant [e.g., amitriptyline (Elavil)], and an anti-Parkinsonism agent [e.g., trihexyphenidyl (Artane)] is freqeuently employed. Each of these agents has a considerably different primary effect; however, all of them possess anticholinergic activity. Even though the anticholinergic effect of any one of the drugs may be slight, the additive effects of the three agents may be significant, resulting in dryness of the mouth, blurring of the vision and other characteristic anticholinergic effects.

Alteration of Gastrointestinal Absorption

1. *Alteration of pH:* Oral dosage forms of the laxative, bisacodyl (Dulcolax), are enteric coated so the drug is not released in the stomach where it could cause significant irritation. It has been suggested that this agent should not be given orally within an hour of antacid (e.g., Gelusil, Maalox) therapy because an increase in the pH of the gastrointestinal contents may cause a disintegration of the enteric coating in the stomach, resulting in the release of bisacodyl in this area which could cause irritation and vomiting.

2. *Complexation:* Tetracycline can combine with metal ions such as calcium, magnesium, aluminum, and iron in the gastrointestinal tract to form complexes that are poorly absorbed. Thus, the administration of certain dietary items (e.g., milk containing calcium) or drugs (e.g., antacids, iron preparations) to patients on tetracycline therapy could cause a significant decrease in the amount of tetracycline absorbed. There is some question as to the extent of the effect of milk on tetracycline absorption and it should be noted that in some instances milk has been given concurrently to help avoid gastrointestinal side effects that frequently accompany the use of the tetracyclines. In these situations the physician may be willing to sacrifice some of the drug's activity in order to have it better tolerated. It is claimed that the absorption of the newest tetracycline, doxyclcine (Vibramycin), is not markedly influenced by the simultaneous ingestion of food or milk and the manufacturer recommends that these substances be given concurrently if gastric irritation occurs. However, the concomitant administration of aluminum hydroxide gel will definitely decrease the absorption of doxycycline.

Stimulation of Metabolism

There are many drugs (e.g., phenobarbital) that are known to increase the activity of liver microsomal enzymes, an effect frequently referred to as enzyme induction. These enzymes are involved in the metabolism of many drugs. For example, it has been shown that the rate of metabolism of the coumarin anticoagulants [e.g., bishydroxycoumarin (Dicumarol), warfarin (Coumadin)] is increased in patients also being treated with phenobarbital. The result of this interaction would be a decreased response to the anticoagulant since it is being more rapidly metabolized and excreted. To compensate for this loss of effect, the dose of the anticoagulant would have to be increased until the desired activity was obtained. Again, a potentially dangerous situation could arise if the patient discontinued taking the phenobarbital and the dose of the anticoagulant was not then appropriately reduced. Such a situation might develop if a hospitalized patient had his warfarin dosage stabilized while he was also receiving phenobarbital. When the patient is discharged from the hospital, there may no longer be a need for the phenobarbital therapy. However, it should be remembered that it may be necessary to change the warfarin dosage when the phenobarbital is discontinued.

Inhibition of Metabolism

A number of cases have been reported where one drug has inhibited the metabolism of a second agent, resulting in a prolonged and intensified activity of the latter. The enzyme, xanthine oxidase, is involved in the metabolism of such potentially toxic drugs as mercaptopurine (Purinethol) and azathioprine (Imuran). When allopurinol (Zyloprim), a xanthine oxidase inhibitor, is given concurrently with one of these agents, the effect of the latter can be markedly increased. It is advised that a reduction in dose to about one-third to one-quarter the usual dose of mercaptopurine or azathioprine will be required when allopurinol is given concurrently. A recent study has indicated that allopurinol can prolong the activity of bishydroxycoumarin by inhibiting its metabolism by liver microsomal enzymes.

Displacement of Drugs from Protein Binding Sites

An interaction of this type may occur when two drugs that are capable of binding to proteins are administered concurrently. Since there are only a limited number of protein-binding sites, a competition will exist and the drug that has the greater affinity for the binding sites will displace the other from plasma or tissue proteins.

Both phenylbutazone (Butazolidin) and warfarin (Coumadin) are bound to plasma proteins. However, apparently phenylbutazone has a greater affinity for the binding sites, resulting in a displacement of the warfarin, making increased quantities of the free drug available. In this situation the activity of the anticoagulant would be increased, possibly resulting in hemorrhaging.

Alteration of Urinary Excretion

1. *Alteration of Urinary pH:* The urinary pH will influence the ionization of weak acids and weak bases and thus affect the extent to which these agents are reabsorbed or excreted. For example, more of an acidic drug will diffuse back into the blood from an acid urine (resulting in a prolonged activity) than from an alkaline urine. The converse will be true for a basic drug like dextroamphetamine (Dexedrine). Studies have shown that the activity of dextroamphetamine can be significantly prolonged when an agent such as sodium bicarbonate, which will increase the pH of the urine, is given concurrently.

2. *Interference with Urinary Excretion:* It is well known that probenecid (Benemid) can increase the serum levels and prolong the activity of penicillin derivatives, by blocking their tubular excretion. This interaction has been used to advantage in the treatment of venereal disease in situations where it was considered preferable to give a large single dose of a penicillin derivative to assure that the patient received all the drug intended. The concurrent administration of probenecid prolongs the activity of this single dose of penicillin.

The potentiation of acetohexamide (Dymelor) hypoglycemia by phenylbutazone (Butazolidin) has been described and it is suggested that phenylbutazone produces this response, in part, by interfering with the renal excretion of hydroxyhexamide, the active metabolite of acetohexamide.

Alteration of Electrolyte Levels

One of the problems associated with the use of many of the newer diuretics is that they produce an excessive loss of potassium. This may present a problem in patients being treated with digitalis derivatives, many of whom would be candidates for diuretic therapy. If a potassium loss remains uncorrected, the heart may become more sensitive to the effects of digitalis and arrhythmia might result. Prolonged therapy with corticosteroids and cathartics may also lead to hypokalemia and cause similar problems.

The use of lithium carbonate (Eskalith, Lithane, Lithonate) has been associated with a number of adverse effects. Since sodium depletion can increase lithium toxicity, it is recommended that the drug should not be used in patients on diuretic therapy or on a sodium-restricted diet.

Interaction at the Adrenergic Neuron

Monoamine oxidase (MAO) functions to break down catecholamines and when it is inhibited, increased levels of norepinephrine within the adrenergic neurons result. Since greater than usual amounts of norepinephrine are now being stored, any drug that might release these stores can bring about exaggerated responses. It is by this mechanism that interactions between monoamine oxidase inhibitors [isocarboxazid (Marplan), nialamide (Niamid), phenelzine (Nardil), tranylcypromine (Parnate), and pargyline (Eutonyl)] and sympathomimetic amines (e.g., amphetamine) develop. Thus, if amphetamine is administered to a patient whose stores of norepinephrine have been increased by MAO inhibition, he may experience severe headache, hypertension (possibly a hypertensive crisis) and cardiac arrhythmias.

Although most sympathomimetic amines, such as amphetamine, are available only by prescription, others such as ephedrine, phenylephrine and phenylpropanolamine are found in many popular non-prescription cold and allergy remedies. Certainly it would be wise for patients being treated with a MAO inhibitor to avoid using products containing these agents.

The tricyclic antidepressants [amitriptyline (Elavil), desipramine (Norpramin, Pertofrane), imipramine (Tofranil), nortriptyline (Aventyl), and protriptyline (Vivactil)] have been known to antagonize the antihypertensive effect of guanethidine (Ismelin), probably by inhibiting the mechanism that concentrates this agent in the neuronal terminal. The newest antidepressant, doxepin (Sinequan), is reported not to block the effects of guanethidine when the dosage of doxepin is less than 100 mg daily.

Although this discussion has been a brief one, it is evident that drug therapy is becoming increasingly complex. The list of drug interactions is a long one and will continue to grow. Those who are involved in drug therapy should be cognizant of potential problems and prepared to prevent their development.

The following list includes selected examples of potential drug interactions that would be of special concern to the podiatrist.

Analgesics and Anti-Inflammatory Agents

Aspirin with

Anticoagulants, e.g., warfarin (Coumadin)

Anticoagulant effect may be increased. Occasional small doses of aspirin will probably not cause difficulty in patients who are well stabilized on anticoagulant therapy; however, aspirin should be given very cautiously and, preferably, not at all to patients in whom there is difficulty in maintaining a constant anticoagulant effect.

Sulfonylurea hypoglycemic agents, e.g. tolbutamide (Orinase)

Effect of the hypoglycemic agent may be enhanced.

Corticosteroids Phenylbutazone (Butazolidin)

Combinations should be used cautiously because of the increased danger of gastrointestinal ulceration.

Indomethacin (Indocin)

Effect of indomethacin may be inhibited; it is suggested that aspirin may impair the gastrointestinal absorption of indomethacin.

Probenecid (Benemid)
Sulfinpyrazone (Anturane)

Aspirin can antagonize the uricosuric activity of these agents. Concurrent therapy should be avoided.

Indomethacin (Indocin) with
  Aspirin

Effect of indomethacin may be inhibited; it is suggested that aspirin may impair the gastrointestinal absorption of indomethacin.

Narcotic analgesics with
  Monoamine oxidase inhibitors, e.g., tranylcypromine (Parnate)

Effect of the narcotic may be enhanced; dosage should be reduced.

  Respiratory depressant drugs, e.g., barbiturates, phenothiazines, etc.

Enhanced respiratory depression may result; dosage of the narcotic should be reduced.

Phenylbutazone (Butazolidin) and Oxyphenbutazone (Tandearil) with
  Oral anticoagulants, e.g. warfarin (Coumadin)

Anticoagulant response may be increased due to displacement of warfarin from protein-binding sites.

  Hypoglycemic agents, e.g., insulin, tolbutamide (Orinase), etc.

Enhanced hypoglycemic effect; phenylbutazone has been reported to interfere with the excretion of the active metabolite of acetohexamide (Dymelor).

  Salicylates, e.g., aspirin

Combinations should be used cautiously because of the increased danger of gastrointestinal ulceration.

Propoxyphene (Darvon) with
  Orphenadrine (Disipal, Norflex)

Mental confusion, anxiety, and tremors have been reported following concurrent use; however, the significance of this potential problem is questionable.

Agents Used in Treating Gout

Allopurinol (Zyloprim) with
  Coumarin anticoagulants, e.g., bishydroxycoumarin (Dicumarol), warfarin (Coumadin)

Allopurinol may inhibit the metabolism of the anticoagulant thereby prolonging its activity.

  Azathioprine (Imuran)

  Azathioprine (Imuran)
  Mercaptopurine (Purinethol)

Allopurinol can inhibit the metabolism of these agents; dose of the agents should be reduced to 1/3 to 1/4 of the usual dose.

Iron salts	Concurrent use should be avoided since an increase in hepatic iron concentration has been reported in animals.
Probenecid (Benemid) with Aminosalicylic acid (PAS)	Probenecid decreases urinary excretion of PAS resulting in increased plasma levels.
Indomethacin (Indocin)	Probenecid interferes with the renal excretion of indomethacin; however, the uricosuric action of probenecid is not blocked.
Penicillin	Probenecid can enhance the effects of penicillin derivatives by interfering with their tubular excretion.
Salicylates, e.g., aspirin	Salicylates antagonize the uricosuric activity of probenecid; concurrent use should be avoided.
Sulfinpyrazone (Anturane) with Citrates, Salicylates	Effect of sulfinpyrazone is antagonized.
Hypoglycemic agents, e.g., insulin, tolbutamide (Orinase), etc.	Hypoclycemic effect may be enhanced.

Corticosteroids*

Corticosteroids (e.g., hydrocortisone, prednisone, triamcinolone) with Diuretics	Excessive potassium depletion may occur since both the corticosteroids and diuretics can cause hypokalemia (potassium depletion).
Hypoglycemic agents, e.g., insulin, tolbutamide (Orinase)	Corticosteroids can cause an increase in blood glucose levels; increased dosage of the hypoglycemic agent may be necessary.
Salicylates	Combinations should be used cautiously because of the increased danger of gastrointestinal ulceration.

Diuretics

Thiazides (e.g., hydrochlorothiazide), chlorthalidone (Hygroton), ethacrynic acid

---

*Problems are not likely to occur when the steroid is applied topically or used locally. However, the use of an occlusive dressing when using a steroid topically increases the possibility of percutaneous absorption and systemic effects. Lower extremity intra-articular injection of steroids may also lead to systemic effects, particularly if superficial veins are accidentally entered.

(Edecrin), furosemide (Lasix) and quinetha-
zone (Hydromox) with
   Corticosteroids

Excessive potassium depletion may occur since these agents and the diuretics can cause hypokalemia.

Digitalis, digoxin, etc.
Digitalis, digoxin, etc.

Diuretics can cause hypokalemia (potassium depletion); if the potassium loss is not corrected the heart can become more sensitive to the effects of digitalis, possibly resulting in digitalis toxicity.

Hypoglycemics, e.g., insulin, tolbutamide (Orinase)

Diuretics can cause an increase in blood glucose levels; increased doses of the hypoglycemic agents may be necessary.

Hypotensive agents, e.g., methyldopa (Aldomet), guanethidine (Ismelin)

Enhanced hypotensive effect; diuretic will frequently permit a reduction in dosage of the hypotensive agent.

Uricosuric agents, e.g., probenecid (Benemid), sulfinpyrazone (Anturane)

Diuretics decrease the renal excretion of uric acid; higher dises of uricosuric agents may be required.

Anti-Infective Agents

Griseofulvin (Fulvicin, Grifulvin, Grisactin)
with
   Coumarin anticoagulants, e.g., warfarin (Coumadin)

Griseofulvin may cause enzyme induction resulting in a more rapid metabolism of the anticoagulant; larger doses of the anticoagulant may be required.

   Phenobarbital

Phenobarbital may decrease the effect of· griseofulvin, possibly by inhibiting its absorption.

Lincomycin (Lincocin) with
   Food, and other drugs

For optimal obsorption, nothing should be given by mouth except water for a period of one to two hours before and after oral administration of lincomycin.

Penicillins with
   Bacteriostatic antibacterials (sulfonamides, tetracyclines, etc.)

Penicillins are bactericidal and only effective against multiplying bacteria; bacteriostatic antibiotics may inhibit their antibacterial effect.

   Food

Penicillins are best absorbed when taken on an empty stomach, at least one hour before or two hours after meals.

Probenecid (Benemid)

Probenecid can enhance the effects of penicillin derivatives by interfering with their tubular excretion.

Tetracyclines with
Anticoagulants

Enhanced anticoagulant effect; response develops, in part, due to interference with the synthesis of Vitamin K by microorganisms in the gastrointestinal tract.

Cations (di- and trivalent such as Ca^{++}, Mg^{++}, and Al^{+++}) in antacids and milk

These cations can combine with the tetracyclines in the gastrointestinal tract to form complexes that are not readily absorbed; a decreased antibiotic effect could result.

Foods

Tetracyclines should be given one hour before or two hours after meals for optimal absorption.

Penicillins

See Penicillins.

Sedative-Hypnotics

Barbiturates (e.g., phenobarbital) with
Alcohol and other central nervous system depressants (narcotics, tranquilizers, etc.)

Enhanced depressant effect.

Oral anticoagulants, e.g. warfarin (Coumadin)

Decreased anticoagulant effect due to enzyme induction; larger doses of the anticoagulant may be required.

Griseofulvin (Fulvicin, Grifulvin, Grisactin)

Decreased effect of griseofulvin; phenobarbital may reduce absorption of griseofulvin.

Monoamine oxidase inhibitors, e.g., tranylcypromine (Parnate)

Effect of barbiturate may be enhance, necessitating a reduction in dosage.

Tranquilizers

Phenothiazines, e.g., chlorpormazine (Thorazine); chlordiazepoxide (Librium); diazepam (Valium); meprobamate (Equanil), etc. with
Central nervous system depressants (alcohol, barbiturates, narcotics, etc.)

Enhanced depressant effect; degree of enhancement depends on the particular tranquilizer used.

Monoamine oxidase inhibitors, e.g., tranylcypromine (Parnate)

MAO inhibitors may enhance the effect of the tranquilizers; an additive hypotensive effect may be seen with the phenothiazines.

Drug Interactions – The Need for Careful History Taking

Samuel Moskow

I must speak as a private clinical investigator, and by this I mean the gauge and standard by which I practice my profession. I have always felt that the foot cannot be separated from the rest of the body. With this in mind, one automatically delves into the practice of medicine in all its aspects.

Several years ago I wrote a letter to the Director of NIH asking the question: "What volunteer services might I offer NIH in the investigation and study of problems of the foot?" The reply to my inquiry was a negative one, with the closing remark in the reply that no investigation was contemplated then or in the future in regard to problems of the foot. So therefore my private clinical studies are the only resource that I have to relate the foot to the other systems of the body which are altered by foot function and pathology.

In my daily practice I treat the mechanical symptoms of the foot first; those of the problems arising from the musculature second; third, the functional and pathologic conditions arising in the osseous system; and fourth, those arising from the variables in the circulation.

As I develop the history along with the treatment of the discomfort of the foot, I constantly investigate the reasons why the foot has presented itself in my office for treatment. As I approach the fifth point that I consider, which medications will aid me in making the foot comfortable. I would like to point out that in many of our problems, usual treatment is doomed to failure unless supplemented by medications, both external and internal. With a background of an oscillometric index, plethysmographic studies, computerized ECG, MSDL approved version for the circulatory apparatus, and a knowledge of the x-ray findings of the feet, I proceed with the routine order of a complete urinalysis and what my laboratory calls a physical examination of the blood.

This physical examination of blood includes the following blood studies: urea and nitrogen; glucose; protein-bound iodine; cholesterol; uric acid; CBC;

Samuel Moskow, D.P.M., *Chairman, APA Council on Podiatric Therapeutics, Washington, D.C.*

and sedimentation rate. I also take the patient's pulse and blood pressure. It is poor medical management to give corticosteroids for any given condition if a patient has a high blood sugar. Massive doses of the salicylates should be avoided if there is a high BUN. With a high cholesterol, any drug of the vasodilator group should be avoided. With the individual with a high uric acid, one must avoid the use of penicillin and the vitamin B preparations. Clinically, if the uric acid is extremely high, one must think of secondary gout associated with a malignancy elsewhere in the body. With a patient with a hypo or hyperthyroid which varies with severe minus or severe plus factor, it would be well for the podiatrist not to prescribe any drugs. With a severe hemoglobin below 10 gm%, one should not operate or prescribe drugs. With a low blood pressure or a high blood pressure, one should proceed cautiously in the prescribing of the vasodilator drugs. The podiatrist, as a member of the healing arts team, must be aware that the art of internal medicine needs to be called upon in order to make the foot problem that has been presented well. He must have the above factors checked and managed on a long-term basis by the internist. Our work in improving the functional capacities of the foot in conjunction with the internal medications will result in a much happier patient. More consultation with the internist would be most enlightening to most podiatrists.

Before proceeding into the assigned topic of the day, let me say this: that the podiatrist should know the drugs that he prescribes well. He should know their adverse reactions as well as their indications. The podiatrist should not prescribe drugs that could create situations that he is unable to manage. The story being: If you cannot handle the adverse reactions that may be caused by any drug, you should not use it. When Dr. Harry Hoffman, former chairman of the Therapeutics Council of the APA and yours truly were assigned the preparation of the Podiatrists' Desk Reference in 1964, this was one of our ground rules as to whether the drug should be utilized in the practice of podiatry. At this point, I would say that we should take to task the statement that podiatrists should be more active in evaluating the clinical efficacy of drugs. This would mean that the major drug houses should utilize the profession in this area of investigation. The pharmaceutical firms do all the fine research on the product. They should establish by the way of grants a rough program of clinical research at the grass roots level in podiatry to answer the question of the drug's advisability and use in daily practice. These rough research links are very important.

The amazing rate of development of new drugs by the pharmaceutical industry and the growing demands of a sophisticated American public for excellence in health care have been accompanied by a significant incidence of previously known and newly recognized forms of drug reactions. While these reactions may involve almost every body organ, the skin appears to be the most frequent target and one where changes are readily recognized by physician and patient alike. In addition to affording the opportunity for easy recognition of drug reactions, the skin, because of its accessibility, is ideal for studying a variety of problems connected with these reactions.

Every new drug has a potential for producing undesirable reactions whether due to overdosage, specific allergic hypersensitivity, or other mechanisms.

Types of Reaction

Cumulative Effects

In order to elicit this type of reaction, prolonged administration of a drug is usually required. Mercurial pigmentation of the nails is well recognized. Patients with psoriasis and seborrheic dermatitis are particularly prone to such pigmentations, possibly because of defective keratin. Hypervitaminosis A, another well-known example, is manifested by thinning, coarsening and loss of hair and localized periosteal swelling. Cumulative effects due to any drug are, of course, particularly likely to become manifest on excessive dosages or upon failure to metabolize or excrete the drug properly. For example, cation toxicity may occur with renal disease or uremia when penicillin is administered in large doses over a short period of time, since 15 million units of potassium penicillin G supplies 25 mEq of potassium.

Pharmacologic Effects

These are due to the expected pharmacologic action of the drug, such as necrosis produced by inadvertent infiltration of extravascular tissues by L-norepinephrine while being administered intravenously.

Overdosage Effects

These are toxic and their occurrence is directly related to the concentration of the drug. The first evidence of overdosage may appear in the skin, as in therapy with anticoagulants where bleeding into the skin is manifested by minute petechiae.

Sanarelli-Shwartzman Reaction

Here it is assumed that the endotoxins elaborated by infectious micro-organisms provide the skin-preparatory factors. The eliciting factor is the antigen-antibody complex consisting of drug plus antibodies to the drug or drug derivative. Certain severe purpuric reactions, such as those due to barbiturates, may be based on this reaction.

Biotropic Effect

This represents activation of a latent or dormant cutaneous infection by a drug. Flares of herpes simplex by barbiturates illustrates this.

Ecologic Imbalance

These reactions are based on disturbances in the normally prevailing balance between different species of microorganisms. An example is overgrowth of monilia in the mouth and anogenital region after therapy with broad spectrum antibiotics or penicillin. Production of glossitis or black hairy tongue following antibiotics may also be explained on the basis of changes in bacterial flora.

Jarisch-Herxheimer Reaction

This is characterized by exacerbation of existing lesions or development of a new eruption following administration of a highly effective drug for an infectious disease. It represents a tissue response to toxic or allergenic products released by the drug-susceptible microorganisms. Fifty percent of patients with syphilis who are treated with penicillin experience this reaction in the form of malaise, fever, and exacerbation of skin lesions 8 to 24 hours following treatment.

Onycholysis seen in patients taking demethylchlortetracycline is an example of a phototoxic type of photosensitivity reaction, while chlorothlazide-type diuretic drugs, which are disulfonamides, have been reported to produce photoallergy but not phototoxicity.

Toxic Epidermal Necrolysis

This syndrome has been described relatively recently. Many cases have been shown to have been caused by drugs. Clinically, the patient may first show small patches of erythema which progress to generalized erythema, in most cases with brawny scaling and bullae with extensive denudation of the skin. It is the complete denudation of the skin over the entire body which is characteristic of this form of drug reaction. Histologically, the epidermis shows necrotic changes in the form of bullae, but there are few, if any, dermal changes. Excellent therapeutic results have been produced with steroids in some patients, but the syndrome is often fulminant and may lead to death from sepsis or electrolyte imbalance as a result of fluid loss from the denuded body surface. Drugs implicated have been penicillin, phenolphtalein, barbiturates, sulfones, sulfonamides and phenylbutazone.

Tumors and Tumor-like Reactions

Both benign and malignant tumors may be produced by drugs. For example, prolonged administration of arsenic in Fowler's Solution and in other medicaments may years later produce warty lesions on the palms and soles which may become squamous cell carcinomas, as well as superficial basal cell epitheliomas, usually found on the trunk.

The question of whether a drug produces a reaction based on an allergic or other mechanism often cannot be readily answered. This is illustrated by the report of polyneuropathy in a child who, after prolonged topical use of ammoniated mercury ointment for insect bites, developed pronounced weakness of leg muscles and an eosinophilia of 9 to 25%.

We have observed a patient with a bullous and epidermal necrolysis-like reaction due to mercury-salicylic ointment used over large skin areas. The eruption responded well to BAL (Dimercaprol); a decision concerning the allergic or toxic nature of the reaction was not possible.

Penicillin is the major single cause of systemic drug reactions in the United States.

In 1961 it was estimated that 100 to 300 deaths due to penicillin occurred annually in the United States. The anaphylactic reaction occurs within seconds or minutes after administration of penicillin to patients previously sensitized either by therapeutic dosages orally or parenterally or by other contact with penicillin, e.g., in dairy products, vaccines and beer. Milk products may contain penicillin when livestock are treated for mastitis, or when the drug is added directly to lower bacterial counts. A quart of milk may contain up to 100 units of penicillin.

The investigators concluded that skin-sensitizing antibody was the most likely candidate for mediating the anaphylactic reaction. When 1,146 patients without history of penicillin allergy were examined, no systemic anaphylactic reactions to penicillin occurred when skin tests with penicilloyl polylysine were negative. The conclusion reached was that a patient with a negative test might develop a subsequent penicillin reaction but it would not be of the immediate anaphylactic type.

Over 1,000 naval recruits were tested for penicillin hypersensitivity. Of these, 825 men with negative skin tests to penicilloyl polylysine showed no anaphylactic reactions to subsequent penicillin administration. Among those with positive skin tests, none developed an anaphylactic reaction to subsequent penicillin therapy, but it is noteworthy that the incidence of urticarial or other skin eruptions was almost ninefold greater in these subjects than in the negative reactors. This study also demonstrated a greater incidence of positive skin reactions in atopic individuals, which fits in with the already known fact that atopic individuals in general have a much greater susceptibility to anaphylactic reactions than do non-atopics. Obviously this is conditioned by the genetic factors which produce the state of atopy. A clinical hypersensitivity state which is subject to hereditary influences would include hay fever, asthma and eczema.

Treatment with another antibiotic is substituted for penicillin in patients with positive skin test reactions. Patients with histories of reactions to penicillin should not be treated with penicillin. However, if patients with past histories of penicillin sensitivity are to be tested, emergency treatment facilities such as epinephrine and oxygen should be immediately available.

Despite these encouraging results, it must be emphasized that further evaluation of the test with penicilloyl polylysine is necesssary before routine usage is advised. It is also possible that in the future additional assessment of the patient's clinical state of sensitization to penicillin will be necessary.

Although anaphylaxis is the most serious penicillin reaction, serum sickness and delayed urticarial lesions are the allergic manifestations of penicillin hypersensitivity most frequently encountered. Serum sickness is characterized by arthralgia, fever, urticaria, often with angioedema or diffuse erythema, proteinuria, lymphadenopathy and, in severe forms, by generalized periarteritis, occurring within several days to weeks after treatment. After an incubation period of sensitization has elapsed, this reaction may occur after only one exposure to penicillin, in contrast to anaphylaxis which occurs only after more than one exposure.

Patients with this kind of reaction are usually benefited by combined administration of corticosteroids and antihistamines. Complete elimination of all sources of penicillin, including foods such as dairy products, is mandatory.

The next most common type of reaction is urticaria occurring within two to 24 hours and up to several weeks after administration of penicillin. The details of its immunologic mechanism have not been adequately delineated. Eosinophilia may be the sole manifestation of a penicillin allergy, or may accompany other signs of allergic penicillin reactions.

Peripheral neuropathy has resulted from the intramuscular use of penicillin, probably from injection immediately into the parenchyma of the nerve.

The practicing podiatrist has a tremendous opportunity and obligation to prevent drug reactions and to assist appropriate organizations and agencies in finding new causes and varieties of drug reactions. This can best be achieved by: 1. prescribing only those drugs which are truly essential to improvement of the patient's foot condition; 2. acquainting himself with the potential of different drugs to produce side effects and to choose those which are least likely to do harm; 3. familiarizing himself with the various known forms of drug reactions, thus being able to recognize such reactions at the earliest possible moment and to immediately discontinue the offending drug or drugs; and 4. being on the alert for new causes and forms of drug reactions not previously recognized so that they may be reported to the appropriate organizations and agencies. This is the great area where the podiatrist can make a contribution.

These efforts, combined with further research in the laboratory and clinic on the mechanism of drug reactions will enable the podiatrist to render far more effective and safer treatment.

The curative value of griseofulvin in mycotic infections of the glabrous skin is also well established, but is far from being as uniform and as satisfactory as in tinea capitis and barbae. Relapses may and do occur after apparent clinical and mycological cure. Such relapses are associated particularly with infections caused by T. rubrum. No acceptable explanation has been yet offered. Either these relapses are due to peculiar immunobiological changes, attributable to certain individuals, or to the production of griseofulvinase. As a possible cause, dysproteinemia has been considered, as well as the production of griseofulvin-resistant strains. It is equally puzzling why interdigital mycoses caused by T. mentagrophytes frequently show a meager response to griseofulvin. This statement is also applicable to a certain degree to the vesicular type of T. mentagrophytes infections of other regions of the glabrous skin.

Regarding treatment of onychomycosis, the keynote is patience. It is undeniable that no cures and relapses occur as well as griseofulvin-resistant cases. Avulsion of nails combined with griseofulvin medication does not appreciably shorten the time of treatment or increase the cure rate. Whether internal medication with biotin (transaminatose protein synthesis CO_2 fixation) increases nail growth, thereby accelerating the deposition of griseofulvin, has as yet not been confirmed. It is, however, an undeniable fact that the thicker the nail plate, the slower the cure rate. This applies to a great extent to the big toe nails. Doubts are expressed that griseofulvin can be as readily traced in all nails as is easily possible on the scalp and in all hair.

Aplasia of infected nails undoubtedly retards the cure. Therefore, organic or spastic vascular changes of the nail matrix not only delay, but also prevent a cure. Griseofulvin therapy may in such instances be combined with the administration of appropriate vasodilators. The aforementioned statements indicate not only a deficiency in our understanding of basic immunological phenomena but also that the pharmacodynamic effect of griseofulvin requires further investigations. These problems posed by griseofulvin may give an added impetus to the solution of many basic problems related to the immunology and therapy of superficial fungus infections.

Toxic Effect

Adverse reactions to the topical application of tolnaftate were not encountered. In massive doses, administered to dogs, the drug did not produce toxic effects. Doses of 0.5 gm/kg daily for 30 consecutive days did not produce abnormalities in external appearance or body weight and there were no gross or microscopic pathologic changes observed at autopsy.

Griseofulvin

In vitro studies proved this drug to be fungistatic against Trichophyton rubrum, T. tonsurans, T. mentagrophytes, T. verrucosum, T. schoenleinii, Microsporum audouinii, M. canis, M. gypseum and Epidermophyton floccosum. It is not effective against bacteria, Candida albicans, or any of the deep fungi.

Clinical Indications

Results are disappointing when the drug is used in the treatment of interdigital infections due to the dermatophytes. It is of no value in the treatment of monilial infections.

Adverse Reactions

Epigastric discomfort, nausea, and diarrhea are the most commonly encountered side effects of oral administration of griseofulvin. Photosensitivity reaction and uticaria are occasionally observed. Patients undergoing griseofulvin therapy should avoid unnecessary exposure to sunlight. Serious adverse reactions have not been encountered.

Anti-rheumatic Diseases

Clinical control of the various rheumatic diseases is dependent to a great extent on empirical therapy with drugs whose action may not be at all clear. To say that a drug has anti-inflammatory or anti-rheumatic activity is almost a play on words, because the mechanism of that action is largely unknown and the observed clinical effect of the drug on inflammation or rheumatic activity is the sole basis for such a designation. For example, colchicine, which has been in use for centuries, is believed to have a specific anti-inflammatory effect in gout, but the actual mechanisms of producing this effect are understood very poorly, if at all. Therefore, in judging the relative values of various anti-rheumatic drugs, one must recognize that such assessment if based largely on clinical evaluation, which by its very nature cannot have sharp delineations or yield precise results – all of which makes drug evaluation difficult and a sometimes frustrating experience.

Although aspirin has long been regarded as indispensable in the treatment of rheumatic disease, there has been an increasing awareness of its irritating and ulcerogenic action of the gastric mucosa. These side effects, together with the unpleasant and often unacceptable (though reversible) tinnitus and deafness, have limited more effective clinical application of salicylates because of the necessity for dosage restrictions.

Prednisone is still the steroid of choice in most patients because it is the least expensive and, generally speaking, produces the fewest complications. However, when prednisone does cause extracellular fluid accumulation or the very occasional idiosyncratic side effect, triamcinolone or dexamethasone may be substituted to advantage. Triamcinolone has potent appetite suppressant action and should be avoided in the underweight patient. In an occasional patient, triamcinolone may cause a general weakness and malaise as well as varying degrees of myasthenia and of potassium deficiency.

Infrequently, dexamethasone may cause considerable extracellular fluid accumulation. Corticosteroids should be prescribed individually and not as a part of a combination tablet, such as with aspirin or phenylbutazone.

Allopurinol

For unknown reasons, attacks of acute gout often occur with increased frequency during the early stages of allopurinol therapy and, therefore, it is wise to start the individual simultaneously on colchicine in a dose of one tablet (0.5 mg) two or three times daily. Continued administration of uricosuric drugs is strongly recommended for the first six months of therapy; afterwards they should no longer be necessary.

Indomethacin

Clinical trials have shown that adverse effects of indomethacin are limited to the cerebral and gastric areas. The cerebral side effects consist of headaches (sometimes quite violent), lightheadedness, unsteadiness, fuzziness and sometimes feelings of detachment; these are transient, disappear promptly on discontinuing the drug and leave no harmful residual effects. These side effects are curiously most common in the morning and can be avoided to a great extent by giving the first dose with lunch and the largest dose at bedtime with milk. The gastric side effects can be avoided by giving the medication on a full stomach and with liberal amounts of milk at bedtime. Isolated cases of dermatitis, somnolence, insomnia, irritable colon and a few other idiosyncratic effects have been observed or reported.

Antibiotics

Continuing the use of an antibiotic when superinfection has appeared is reprehensible because it perpetuates the circumstances under which the new organism has been able to establish a pathogenic hold. Failure to stop administration of a given antibiotic when certain types of reaction appear is also an abuse. The following reactions should warn the physician of danger: an anaphylactoid reaction, thrombopenia, severe leukopenia, hemolytic anemia, disturbance of vestibular or auditory function, evidence of renal insufficiency, serum sickness, angioneurotic edema, exfoliative dermatitis and purpura. Failure to make searching inquiry into the possibility that the patient may have experienced a previous reaction to the drug that is to be used is certainly a dereliction of duty and therefore an abuse. And finally, the use of certain antibiotics without definite knowledge that the patient is free of renal disease; the only antibiotics that can be used safely in full dosage in an individual with severe renal failure are chloramphenicol, erythromycin, noboviocin and chlortetracycline. Even the dosage of penicillin must be reduced in a patient with renal insufficiency.

Thiamine HCl

Several reports have appeared of an anaphylactic type of reaction in patients apparently sensitized by repeated injections of thiamine. Skin tests are fairly reliable in detecting thiamine sensitivity, the scratch being superior to the intradermal test. Symptoms resembling those of hyperthryroidism have also been reported, and it has often been observed that thiamine administration is followed by an unexplained transitory increase of riboflavin excretion in the urine.

Nicotinamide does not cause any deleterious effects, but nicotinic acid, in addition to the flushing which manifests its selective vasodilator action, sometimes causes urticaria, nausea and vomiting, occasionally circulatory collapse or a severe anaphylactic reaction, the two latter occurrences being associated with intravenous administration. Many persons have had a slight elevation in blood sugar and a positive glucose tolerance test, both also reversible.

Coumarins

Both potentiation and inhibition of anticoagulant activity have been observed in patients taking other drugs along with coumarin anticoagulants. Coumarins can also affect the activity of other drugs. No method is available for predicting the occurrence or degree of interaction. Its extent may vary greatly from patient to patient, mainly because of differences in rate of metabolism; interactions have, in some cases, been serious enough to cause death.

Some drugs increase microsomal enzyme activity in the liver, thus stimulating metabolic degradation of the coumarins and reducing their anti-coagulant effect: patients are then likely to need larger amounts of anticoagu-lant, and when the drugs are discontinued, the dose of the anticoagulant may have to be reduced. The drugs most clearly implicated in reports of such interactions are phenobarbital and chloral hydrate; other drugs with a potential for microsomal enzyme stimulation include other barbiturates, meprobamate and griseofulvin.

Potentiating effects may also occur with drugs that displace the anticoagu-lant from protein binding sites in plasma, thus greatly increasing the peak concentration of free coumarin. Drugs having this effect include salicylates.

Tetracyclines, neomycin, and possibly other antibiotics may prolong prothrombin time in patients on oral anticoagulant drugs, mainly by interference with vitamin K production by gut bacteria. Quinine and quinidine also increase the anticoagulant effects of coumarin though the mechanisms are unclear.

Photosensitivity

Among the numerous systemic drugs known to cause photosensitivity reactions are the sulfonamides (antibacterial, thiazide, and hypoglycemic), tetracyclines, griseofulvin (Grisactin, Grisfulvin V, Fulvicin-U/F), and some phenothiazines, barbiturates and salicylates.

The topical agents most frequently responsible for photosensitivity reactions are the halogenated salicylanilides. These antiseptic agents are present in Cuticura, Lifebuoy, Phase III, Safeguard, Zest and other soaps. Photosensitivity reactions may also occur with other antiseptics contained in deodorant soaps.

Photosensitivity reactions are usually characterized by erythematous, vesicular, papular or eczematous lesions. The reaction may persist for prolonged periods without further contact with the sensitizing agent. The primary therapy is elimination of the photosensitizing agent or restriction of exposure to sunlight.

Corticosteroid Joint Injection

Intra-articular (intrasynovial) administration of corticosteroids in joints affected by rheumatoid arthritis or osteoarthritis has been used most often where systemic steroid therapy has been ineffective or could not be tolerated, or where symptoms have been limited to a few large joints. Clinicians differ, however, as to the effectiveness of such therapy, and some who accept its effectiveness doubt that the benefits are great enough to justify the hazards.

J. L. Hollander has reported improvement lasting for at least a few days following intrasynovial injection of steroids in several thousand patients with rheumatoid arthritis or osteoarthritis. Other clinicians have reported success in from 50 to 80% of patients. Some clinicians have reported success in steroids useful in osteoarthritis but not in rheumatoid arthritis; others have found such therapy useful in rheumatoid arthritis but not osteoarthritis. Rheumatoid arthritis in particular is subject to spontaneous remission of unpredictable duration, with emotional factors often influencing the course of the disorder. Study of the effectiveness of drug therapy, especially when uncontrolled, is therefore difficult, and contradictory results in different trials not unexpected.

Intra-articular steroids are most likely to be temporarily helpful in joints in which there is effusion. The reported improvement in symptoms and in objective findings generally occurs within 48 hours and it may persist for a few days to a month.

Adverse Effects

Although there have been reports on patients who have had frequent treatment with intra-articular steroids for as long as 15 years without apparent ill effect, such therapy is often associated with destructive joint changes. Even when they appear to have beneficial effects, steroids cannot prevent the degeneration of cartilage which is characteristic of osteoarthritis, and there is experimental evidence that they actually inhibit protein synthesis in articular cartilage. Depression of cartilage metabolism may be a factor in the development of the Charcot-type of joint disorder. The joint should not be used. All of this is quoted from the authentic Medical Letter. My personal experience with the corticosteroids, having used hydrocortisone acetate ever since it became commercially available on the market, has not substantiated this finding. I have on file over 40,000 x-rays that would substantiate this finding. I question the validity of this statement.

Joints that are infected, severely deformed, or unstable should not be treated by intra-articular therapy.

A transient flare-up of symptoms is seen in about 2% of injected joints. This reaction usually occurs within two or three hours after injection and resolves spontaneously within 24 hours. Systemic absorption of steroids from injected joints does occur, but there is no evidence that adrenal suppression is a clinical problem with a limited number of intra-articular injections of small doses.

YOU ALONE SHALL BE THE JUDGE OF WHAT TO CONDEMN AND WHAT TO AGREE TO. You are like the President of the United States, the buck stops when you prescribe. You must prescribe only those drugs whose actions, interactions and adverse reactions you know. What you say to your patient when you hand the prescription to him is as important as the drug that you prescribe. Take advantage of this important catalyst, the power of suggestion, when you prescribe.

The Management of Reactions to Local Anesthetics

S. Crawford Duhon

Twenty to forty years ago sensitivity reactions to injected local anesthetics were seldom recognized. Those of us encountering them were inclined to feel that these women (it almost always was a female) had "the vapors."

There were several reasons for this failure to appreciate what was happening. One was that there was inconsistence of reaction to such anesthetic agents. A previous reaction failed to materialize the next time, so that many clinicians felt that there was no such thing as a bona fide reaction to an injected anesthetic.

Personally, I feel that the vast majority of such responses are of the nature of cumulative reactions. That is that several exposures in a relatively short period (for instance weekly for 3 or more times) are responsible.

Many dentists are aware of this relationship and avoid giving appointments more frequently than once monthly.

However, fixed reactions do exist — where the usage at any time of the product will invariably produce clinical signs and symptoms of varying degrees of severity. In some instances the reaction can be life threatening.

These reactions are well known to all of us — signs of collapse with low blood pressure, weak thready pulse, perhaps with pulse irregularities, pallor, sweaty, cool skin with accompanying symptoms of feeling faint, palpitation, shortness of breath and peculiar sensations of numbness and tingling far beyond the anaesthetized areas.

The amount of anesthetic producing such a response in such cases is not due to excessive dosage — it occurs with a small dose, regardless of how small.

My goal is to describe a method of both preventing or rapidly clearing such reactions which you each can readily perform on these cases in your office.

In my opinion, it would be best to accomplish prophylactic neutralization, as these reactions, while frightening to both the patient and the surgeon or clinician, are potentially disruptive of the planned surgical procedure.

S. C. Duhon, M.D., *Director, American Society of Clinical Ecology, Boulder, Colorado.*

Dr. R. H. Richardson, also of Boulder, was instrumental in my appearance on this panel of drug reactions. I am no authority on drugs and their reactions, but I have been a general practitioner for some thirty years, who has been drawn increasingly into a practice of allergy or more correctly clinical ecology – allergy and chemical sensitivities.

In December of 1970, Dr. Richardson called upon me to see such a patient. She had received 1-1/2 cc's of 1% Xylocaine plain. She reacted within 2 minutes. He gave the patient Decadron, 4 mg/cc in divided doses of 2 mg each, concurrently with 1 cc Dimetane 100 mg/cc. All to no avail.

We are in the same building, so in a matter of minutes I had returned to my office and obtained several dilutions of a 1% Xylocaine solution. After taking her pulse, I used a tuberculin syringe to remove 0.05 cc of the #1 dilution of Xylocaine and then dropped it under her tongue, cautioning her not to swallow it. In a very few moments she volunteered that she felt better.

After again taking her pulse, I similarly administered the same amount out of the #2 bottle. These are 1:5 dilutions of the Xylocaine. In 1-1/2 to 2 minutes after the second drop she reported that she now felt quite normal. Dr. Richardson went ahead and did the surgery on one foot with the additional use of 1 cc of 1% Xylocaine with no reaction whatsoever. Later, she came back and had the surgery on the other foot. Prior to this second use of the anesthetic we tested her and produced a mild reaction with the same amount of one or two dilutions and then neutralized this with another dilution. She had no effect from the use of the Xylocaine as the anesthetic agent, the day following the neutralization.

I shall describe the preparation of such dilutions in detail as well as give directions for neutralizing such reactions, but first let me supply a bit of historical background:

In 1960, one Carleton Lee, a pediatrician assuming an allergy practice in St. Joseph, Missouri, was under the tutelage of the late Herbert J. Rinkel of Kansas City, Missouri. Dr. Lee wished to relieve symptoms produced by the then effective method of testing foods – the Deliberate Feeding Test of Rinkel.

The test was painfully slow as a food had to be totally avoided for a minimum of four days. It then was tested singly on the fifth day. Another food could be tested the next day if the symptoms had not been too severe and had subsided with the help of a saline laxative.

Dr. Lee wished to remove the symptoms thus produced in order to make it possible to test more than one food in a single day. Dr. Rinkel instructed him in the preparation of food extracts and was, I am sure, surprised when Dr. Lee began to neutralize the symptoms. Dr. Rinkel immediately knew that symptoms could as well be provoked – a test performed – with the use of more than one dilution injected into or under the skin. Several allergists some 35 years before, including Drs. Ethan Allen Brown, Lovelace, and Rinkel, had failed in provoking symptoms with single injections. (personal communication Herbert J. Rinkel, 1961.)

Dr. Lee has evolved a very effective intradermal technique since that 1960 beginning. However I shall leave the intradermal and subcutaneous routes to discuss the sublingual method as I feel it more applicable to chemicals and better suited for the use of this specialty group.

Briefly, in 1949, I had been privileged to see Dr. Rinkel relieve an asthmatic in the course of an hours presentation of the use of "high dilution technique" (autumn pollens). Therefore, I sought his help when I myself developed asthma in 1957 and began the study of allergy under his tutelage at both formal seminars and in the course of a close friendship and association that lasted until his death in 1963.

He had demonstrated the subcutaneous provocative test to me in 1961 in my office and I used it exclusively until 1963 when I began the use of the sublingual route as a medium of provocative testing. Dr. French Hansel, an ENT allergist from St. Louis, Missouri, had used the under the tongue route for years to administer antigens such as dust and molds.

It was not until the first of this year that I have again returned to the use of a refined intradermal technique (C. Lee) for the provocative testing, but more particularly for neutralization of food reactions. I still prefer the sublingual approach for neutralization of medications.

We, like many others using either of the two routes of provocation, confirmed what Carleton Lee stated early in his experience with the intradermal provocative test, that the weaker dilutions of an antigen produced the stronger clinical reactions and that neutralization should be best attempted with the stronger dilutions of the antigen or chemical incitant.

Also, we agree that skipping about in the selection of dilutions is less productive of the establishment of good neutralization dosages than methodical 1 dilution progression.

First, I will list the necessary materials for making these simple dilutions:

Several dozen 5 cc glass vials and rubber stoppers to fit them
3 cc Disposable syringes with 21 gauge needles or
2 cc Leur-Lock syringes
Tuberculin type syringes with 27 gauge needles
Labels for proper identification of each dilution
Index cards for recording dilutions used and any reaction to specific dilutions and pulse readings
Coca's extracting solution consisting of a mixture of
     5 gms. Sodium Chloride
   2.5 gms. Sodium Bicarbonate
     2 liters Sterile Water for Injection

If you would rather not bother with sterilizing bottles after capping them, these can be purchased already prepared from allergy supply houses, such as a local outlet:

> Meridian Bio-Medical, Inc.
> 3278 S. Wadsworth
> Denver, Colorado 80227
> Telephone (303) 985-2111

Questions and Comments

Moderator: John R. Graham

MODERATOR: Thank you very much, Dr. Duhon. I am going to throw this meeting open to questions from the floor. However, I have made some observations. I think I will question directly some of the panel members myself before I open up the meeting to questions from the audience. There is one bit of information that I would like to give you. I would like to tell you of a booklet prepared by Dr. Hussar for Lederle. I think that if you will contact Lederle and ask them to mail you a copy of *Methods of Drug Interactions,* you will find this to be a most valuable addition to your clinical prowess. I think this is something that everybody should have and read. It goes into far more detail than Dr. Hussar had the time to do this morning. I would like to go back to you, Dr. Duhon, regarding reactions to local anesthetics. As we know, all local anesthetics are central nervous system stimulants. I am wondering what relationship we are actually talking about as far as pharmacological effects are concerned and physiological effects are involved. Individuals being alarmed, worried psychogenically, have an elevated blood pressure, they kick out a little bit more adrenalin merely being psychogenically induced. We come along and we give them our local anesthetics to which we have added a vaso-constrictor. Would the method that you mentioned have any effect on this type of reaction, which is actually a reaction of the central nervous system? Is that question stated clearly enough for you?

DR. DUHON: I find it difficult to limit my answer because of several factors. First, let me say that in the case we were talking about, of course, we had no epinephrine in the anesthetic. I think that many of these so-called

---

John R. Graham, D.P.M., *Board of Trustees, American Podiatry Association, Decatur, Illinois.*

reactions or supposed reactions to the epinephrine are not that at all. But they are to sensitivity reactions. Sensitivity reactions produce psychiatric neurological disorders, symptomatology, as it were. But this is not written by our group. There is a book on *Neurology and Psychiatric Disorders Due to Allergy* and the author is an allergist, whose name escapes me at the moment, who is connected with the University of Missouri Medical School in Kansas City, Missouri. The contributors to the book are neurologists from all over the country and psychiatrists from all over the country. Reactions to drugs are very prevalent as causes of neurological and psychiatric disorders. This brings to mind my own experience. When I got out of the service I had had one year in New York City, a residency half at Columbia University and half at a mental hospital in New York City. I was psychiatrically oriented to the extent that my asthmatic patients were sent to a good psychiatrist here in Denver. I practice in Boulder, Colorado, in case you don't remember. We did not help these patients to solve their asthmatic problem. As you know, many people feel that bronchial asthma is due to psychological factors. These patients were helped in their interpersonal relationships. I feel that this is the same sort of misconception that we have about many reactions as being due to appre-hension, that occurs with local anesthetics. I feel that it must be proven that the small amount of epinephrine that is used is producing the overall effect because of its pharmacologic effect. Is it the epinephrine? Or is it the anesthetic itself that is producing a sensitizing reaction? That gives you the rapid heart beat, irregularities of pulse, apprehension, and everything else that goes with it. Of course, when you are in shock, I am sure that you have a lot of apprehension about the outcome.

MODERATOR: Thank you, Dr. Duhon. I would like to direct this question to Dr. Hussar. One of the things that we as podiatrists very fre-quently encounter are individuals who are on thiazides, particularly diuretics. One of the interesting sidelights we see with this is the hyperuricemia. Whether we are dealing with a chemical gout or a true gout, sometimes it can be treated as such with symptomatic relief. My question to you Dr. Hussar, is through what mechanism do we get this hyperuricemia. This apparently is not appreciated as much by doctors of medicine as it is by doctors of podiatry. My specific question to you, Dr. Hussar, is there any way of depressing that uricemia? What mechanism should be used?

DR. HUSSAR: I am not aware of an exact mechanism by which this effect occurs. I do not feel that it has been well defined. However, it is recognized, as you point out, that this definitely is a possibility with the thiazides and also with the related diuretics in that there can be hyperuricemia developing. Apparently certain patients are more susceptible to this than others. Patients who already have gout: it might certainly be expected that this might aggravate their condition. This might necessitate an increase in the dose of uricosuric agents such as Benemid or one of the others. But as far as the specific mechanism, I can't give a solid answer. I don't feel that a definitive mechanism has been established, to have the thiazide produce an increase in the uric acid level.

MODERATOR: Dr. Hussar, more specifically on reactions and inter-reactions, one of the drugs that we very frequently use, as Dr. Moskow touched upon, is Griseofulvin. Would you mention some of the effects it might have upon anticoagulants?

DR. HUSSAR: The two interactions which have been reported with Griseofulvin were touched upon in my presentation – one was phenobarbital. Phenobarbital could decrease the effect of Griseofulvin. Griseofulvin, as Dr. Graham suggests, has also been known to react with anticoagulants. And it is suggested that Griseofulvin may decrease the response to anticoagulants such as coumadin or dicumerol. The suggested mechanism here is that Griseofulvin may have some ability to increase the activity of the liver enzymes in a manner similar to the one we discussed with phenobarbital. In this manner it may decrease the effect of the anticoagulant.

MODERATOR: I made an observation as Dr. Hussar was going through some of the various interreactions. He talked of duccolax and the change in alteration of the pH of the gastric contents. There are so many readily available antacids over the counter it clearly points to the glaring necessity – and I am satisfied Dr. Duhon appreciates this more than we do – of the need for some classification and control of medication. You will be happy to know that your American Podiatry Association in conjunction with the American Pharmaceutical Association has tried to lend what support they can in achieving this legislation on both the national and state and local levels. There has to be some control over the amount of drugs that individuals are securing at liberty in drug stores or food shops or grocery stores. If we have emphasized one thing, it is the need for this control. It is becoming glaringly apparent that the practitioner has to know what other medication his patient is taking before he deems it necessary to add to that amount of medicine.

(QUESTION FROM AUDIENCE:) Is there any available knowledge or material relating to the incorporation of Erythromyocin in an anesthetic base? I allude to the combination of penicillin with an anesthetic base? I also allude to a combination of penicillin with a procaine base.

DR. HUSSAR: I am not aware of any specific published studies dealing with this problem. Of course, procaine penicillin is probably one of the most long standing examples of such a combination. This continues to be widely used on an intramuscular basis to obtain a sustained effect of the penicillin. The reason for including a local anesthetic and some of the other antibiotic formulations is, of course, to decrease the pain on intramuscular injection. Drugs like Erythromycin and Coly-mycin have been marketed in formulations that include a local anesthetic. I think some of the tetracycline intramuscular formulations also do this. I think that where possible there is a trend away from this, possibly as a result of reports such as you have mentioned. I can't recall having seen any of these reports. Keflin is another drug. I don't think Keflin comes formulated with a local anesthetic but I think one of Lilly's suggestions is that, because Keflin, when injected I.M. can cause pain, it might be mixed with something like procaine.

MODERATOR: I would say that Dr. Hussar mentioned Keflin. You might go to Lilly and ask them to tell you about Keflex, which is an oral antibiotic not of the same structure but of the same effect.

(QUESTION FROM AUDIENCE:) What would be our first step in case we encounter a reaction with a local anesthetic after injection? I would like Dr. Duhon to answer.

DR. DUHON: I think that if the reaction were severe for medicolegal reasons I would follow the usual recommendation of using the steroid and perhaps a decongestant, particularly adrenalin. And if you still had difficulty, I would proceed immediately to use 0.05 cc of a Number 1 vial if you already had it made up. If you don't have it made up, it would take you just a few minutes to make it up if you had all of the equipment available to you. It would only take one minute to make your dilutions out to Number 6. Then I would go to this procedure. I would use 0.05 cc of the Number 1 vial under the tongue, having taken the pulse, and then proceed to the Number 2, and the Number 3. Unless conditions were worsening, in which case I would not be afraid to use the concentrate if this was the case. I would use 0.05 cc of the strength that gave the reaction. This procedure works very rapidly and it is very dramatic to see it work. And it does work! We do not see many cases of this but we use it all the time. Let me digress a bit. We have had a large experience with this, we use it for medications on our allergy patients who must take such things as eye medications that an ophthalmologist will wish his patient to be on and when they are well-controlled they are on an ecological management, that is, their chemicals in their environment are minimized. And these people will react very obviously to chemicals that are still in their environment. Therefore, very shortly you will see that they are having reactions to this medication or that medication or to toothpaste or whatever comes into their environment. The chemicals are then taken out. Therefore, we will neutralize these medications one by one and get rid of the symptoms that the patient is having due to these chemicals. Some of these reactions are very severe. But I can't think of one that we haven't been able to neutralize with medications. Chemicals of this sort, that the patient is taking, respond very well to neutralization. I have gotten away from phenolized extracts because phenol – which is ubiquitous – is everywhere in our environment; in our plastics, in synthetics, in tin can linings, in cans for the packaging of fruits. All of these contain phenolized resins. Phenol is everywhere – in Lysol, in mouthwashes, etc. The ecologist who is getting his patients on ecological management is finding that they are having more and more reactions to phenols. So we have gotten away from phenols. Phenol is not readily neutralized in such cases. This is the one exception. But for medications that we have neutralized for our patients, I can't think of any that we haven't been able to neutralize with very dramatic results. One of my nurses, who has been with me for a year, was with me one day in the examining room. The technician was busy with a group of patients. The technician was at capacity. So I brought in this nurse. I took in a patient – this woman is 85 years old – who I have been treating since I first started practicing in Boulder in 1945. We had her on phenobarbital for years. This woman, incidentally, does not have much allergy to phenobarbital but she does have allergy to many, many other medications. She has hypertension. Through the years we have tried to give her many antihypertensive agents, all with the same result – she would not tolerate them. Recently we had her on an allergy regimen because of her asthmatic cough-prednisolone allergy but she, as a woman, is also on other medications. At age 85. And her ophthalmalogist has her on vascular drugs. We felt that the arthritis that was afflicting her arthralgia in her knee and the myalgia and the headaches and the vertigo were due to these medications. She was in a very bad way. Therefore we took her off and let her go on one medication at a time and then after having been on it for about a week we would bring her in and establish a neutralizing dose. We were doing this for one of her medications, I have forgotten which one. She came in one day from the waiting room, the nurse helped her into the examining room where I performed the sublingual testing and it took her 5 minutes on crutches to get from the waiting room to the examining room, which is about the length of this section of tables here. She was in exquisite pain. Her knee was held straight out on the examining table. It had to be braced. And after the first dilution of the Number 1, she was able to bend her leg and told the nurse so, and after the third one, she said, "I am going home." And she hopped down from the table, carried her crutches out, and the nurse said: "You know, I always thought allergy was a bunch of bologna until I saw this!" But these work very well. As I have said, we have had no failures with the use of this technique.

MODERATOR: Dr. Duhon, I wonder if you can remember any books, any publications that we might better acquaint ourselves with, that covers this particular form of therapy?

DR. DUHON: *The Archives of Otolaryngology* in 1968 carried this technique under the authorship of Doctors Carleton Lee, Edward Binkley, and several others. If you people who are interested will write me a letter, possibly I can secure other reprints for you.

V. Pre- and Post-Operative Biomechanical Considerations in Foot Surgery

Biomechanics and Its Relationship to Foot Surgery

Fritz A. Moeller

Introduction

Biomechanics is known as the application of mechanical laws to living structures and specifically to the locomotor system of the human body. The opportunity to apply these mechanical laws comes as a result of the evolutionary development of our body form.

Certain standard relationships are now recognized as being normal at this stage of our morphogenesis. These normal musculoskeletal relationships come into play in both the static and the functional attitudes.

These musculoskeletal relationships maintain the whole and its various parts in specific attitudes that we call the upright posture. The various osseous elements are intended to undergo specific ranges of motion and to influence and be influenced by specific muscles exerting specific tensions or lack of tensions, the result of which we recognize as the normal gait cycle. The importance of this upright posture and its inherent ability of movement or propulsion is basic to the development and emergence of the homo sapiens.

Both the static and the functional relationships undergo developmental change as the individual human is maturing, and because of this ontogeny, normal values may vary within different age groups. We assume, however, that once the individual has passed the age of puberty, this musculoskeletal developmental history is complete.

Biomechanical Abnormalities

Obviously, there is opportunity for abnormalities to occur. Most of these abnormalities probably represent an arrest in the ontogenetic development, but an individual can also be subject to non-genetic and even emotional influences. When any of these abnormalities do occur, we observe certain clinical manifestations, the specific clinical manifestation is dependent upon the degree of the abnormality, the level at which the abnormality occurs, whether it is

---

Fritz A. Moeller, D.P.M., *Doctors Hospital, Albuquerque, New Mexico.*

structural or functional, whether it is compensated or uncompensated, and whether it is occurring solitarily or in combination with one or more additional abnormalities. When a variety of these factors are coming into play, one must weigh their various synergistic and antagonistic influences and attempt to determine the end result or net effect or, more practically, its most important net effect.

Directing our comments to a specific abnormality and a specific clinical manifestation, plantar lesions of the internal lesser metatarsal heads caused by forefoot varus, how does one practically apply known biomechanical principles when considering the pre- and post-operative management of such a problem?

The Role of the Gait Cycle

First, consider the normal gait cycle as it consists of the stance phase and the swing phase. The swing phase can be simply defined as that portion of the gait cycle when the foot is *not* on the ground, and the stance phase can be defined simply as that greater portion of the gait cycle during which the foot *is* on the ground. During the first 25% of the stance phase of gait the foot is found in a pronated attitude and is undergoing a pronatory motion. This pronation is normal and allows for the unlocking of the midtarsal joint and subtalar joint to act as a shock absorber, to adjust to any irregularities of the weight-bearing surface, and to allow the superimposed leg to undergo internal rotation. During the remaining 75% of the stance phase, the foot is undergoing a supinatory motion with its objective being a fully supinated position of the foot for stability – that is, a rigid lever for mechanical advantage during propulsion. We don't find the foot in an actual supinated position, however, until the second half of the stance phase because the portion between 25% and 50% (mid-stance) is spent recovering from the maximum pronated attitude of normalcy. The superimposed leg reverses its rotary motion at the end of this normal pronatory portion of the stance phase and is externally rotating throughout the last 75% of the time the foot is on the ground.

The Role of the Subtalar and Midtarsal Joints

Supination is defined as inversion, adduction, and plantar flexion. Pronation is defined as eversion, abduction, and dorsiflexion. The subtalar joint possesses the capability of movement in all three planes. The neutral subtalar joint is defined as that position of normalcy wherein the subtalar joint is neither supinated nor pronated. The subtalar joint controls the midtarsal joint, i.e., when it is in its neutral position and the midtarsal joint is maximally pronated (as found at mid-stance), the midtarsal joint is locked or stable. In stance as the subtalar joint supinates, the midtarsal joint pronates. The converse is true but the supination of the midtarsal joint is relative. That is to say, when the subtalar joint is neutral and the midtarsal joint is maximally pronated, the forefoot is perpendicular to the rearfoot. When the subtalar joint is pronated and the midtarsal joint, therefore, unlocked and the foot placed on the supporting surface, the forefoot is inverted relative to the rearfoot because of the eversion of the rearfoot in pronation, but the forefoot is also parallel with the weight-bearing surface.

The Role of Pronation

To return to the practical application of this information: plantar lesions of the internal lesser metatarsal heads occur because of abnormal stresses occurring during the stance phase of gait, and if the foot is pronating at any time during the last 75% of this stance phase of gait instead of supinating or if it is found in a static pronated attitude instead of a supinated attitude during the last 50% of the stance phase of gait, abnormal forces (shear) will occur at the internal lesser metatarsal heads and *excessive* pronation from any cause results in hypermobility of the forefoot.

Three of the more common causes for pronation to be present or to be taking place at a time or segment of the stance phase, when it should not, are compensating varus deformities of the subtalar and midtarsal joints, equinus at the level of the ankle, and hypermobility of the first ray. Theoretically, if one can mechanically control or eliminate this poorly timed pronation, he can improve and even eliminate lesser metatarsal head plantar lesions. This author has frequently found this to occur, not just theoretically, but very, very practically.

The Role of Surgery

If these mechanical means are found to be unsuccessful and the lesion persists, a surgical approach should be considered. Choice of surgical procedure should be made only after thorough understanding of the biomechanics involved and only after establishing post-operative goals for the control of any biomechanical abnormalities. Previously popular surgical approaches for this problem have not produced the consistent satisfactory results we desire.

A more biomechanically logical surgical approach to these lesions is indicated. This surgical procedure should be designed to allow a lessening in the angle of declination and, when indicated, a shortening of the involved metatarsal. The purpose of this type of approach would be to relieve the shearing forces concentrated at the metatarsal head while at the same time avoiding the destruction of a most useful component of the skeletal framework of the foot, the metatarsophalangeal joint. Function of the metatarsophalangeal joint is thus preserved.

Such a surgical approach can be achieved by performing either an extension wedge osteoarthrotomy of the metatarsocuneiform joint or a dorsal wedge osteotomy of the metatarsal base.

Other Local Biomechanics Involving the Internal Lesser Metatarsal Heads

Basically, when considering the biomechanics of this area one must direct comments and attention in two separate categories, the first being the static situation and the second, of course, the functional situation.

Forefoot in Static Stance

In considering the static situation, we must realize that there are three basic forces acting upon the joint and/or bone under consideration: the active force of body weight, the reactive force of gravity, and the force of muscle activity. A second basic premise to be established is the understanding that osseous contributions to the static stability are of more importance than soft tissue contributions.

The plantar forefoot plane parallels the plantar plane of the heel during normal static stance and the plantar plane of the forefoot is perpendicular to the sagittal plane of the calcaneus. The plantar forefoot plane parallels the floor with all five metatarsal heads bearing weight, each internal metatarsal carries an equal distribution of the weight load. The midtarsal joint is locked in a maximum pronated position and no metatarsal or midtarsal motion is possible as long as the subtalar joint remains neutral, metatarsals two, three, and four are locked in their maximum position of dorsiflexion by the reactive force from the floor.

The Forefoot In Function

The primary function of the ligaments associated with the metatarsophalangeal joints in question is to act as a "stop-check" in the event of sudden or unguarded motion. Static stability is a secondary function. Muscles have some effect in this area but, of course, this effect is primarily on the associated phalanges. Consideration should be given, however, to the interossei and the lumbricales as the most pertinent.

Additional factors to consider are the declination angle of the metatarsal itself, keeping in mind that this is variable, it will become increased on supination and decreased on pronation. Also, keep in mind the respective axis of motion of each metatarsocuneiform joint articulation. For instance, the second metatarsal dorsi- and plantar-flexes close to a parallel with the sagittal plane, but the fourth metatarsal dorsi- and plantar-flexes much more oblique to this sagittal plane.

Another biomechanical principle dictates that the greater the angle of adductus of the metatarsus, the more lateral will be the involved metatarsal head.

Also, as the foot pronates, the metatarsals are thrust anteriorward (foot is elongated) with the greatest excursion by the second metatarsal, less by the third, and actually minimal by the fourth.

The second internal metatarsal motion taking place on the transverse plane during pronation is in an abductory direction. The second, again, undergoes the most marked excursion of the lesser metatarsals, but the fourth metatarsal is in motion to a slight abductory degree also.

Frontal plane motion occurs at the metatarsal head by inverting, relatively, during pronation and if one will inspect the metatarsal head of a handy foot model, it is noted that the lateral plantar condyle is probably markedly larger than the medial and during pronation may thus be brought into plantar prominence by the relative axial rotation of the internal lesser metatarsal.

Using the longitudinal axis of the second metatarsal, the first metatarsal deviates from it in an adductory direction. The lateral three metatarsals flare away from the second metatarsal and from each adjacent medial metatarsal in an abductory direction.

Forefoot Varus

The forefoot varus deformity is a fixed congenital osseous deformity and is of prime consideration in this discussion. Forefoot varus is described as having the plantar of the forefoot inverted (directed toward the mid-line of the body) relative to the plantar of the rearfoot when the subtalar joint is neutral and when the midtarsal joint is pronated to its maximum. This author would, however, like to first mention the situation which I prefer to call "functional" forefoot varus. There is hypermobility of the first ray and on a measurement from the first to the fifth metatarsal head, a varus relationship to the rearfoot is obtained. The medial pillar of the weight-bearing "tripod" is absent and allows the foot to essentially fall into a pronated attitude until the extreme of the dorsiflexion range is reached by the first metatarsal or the second metatarsal becomes influential. To repeat, development of first ray hypermobility in a former forefoot valgus tends to cause a "functional" fully compensated varus.

First ray hypermobility usually leads to the formation of callous type lesions under the second metatarsal head and sometimes under both the second and third. These can be well-circumscribed or dispersive. Occasionally, a solitary lesion under the third head occurs and on inspection of the dorsi-plantar x-ray view, the long axis of this third metatarsal may be directed toward the second metatarsal rather than abducted or directed away from it. It is felt that this represents plantar flexion or the so-called increase in declination of the third metatarsal. A fourth metatarsal head lesion may be due to a hypermobile and/or subluxed fifth ray associated with a partially compensated forefoot varus and thus causing the fourth to receive the brunt of the weight stresses as they pass forward along the lateral side of the foot.

Additional Factors

Because hammer toes are commonly seen in the compensated forefoot varus abnormality, the retrograde force of the proximal phalanx upon the dorsum of the metatarsal head when the deformed forefoot is placed in a shoe may sometimes contribute to the etiologic mechanism of plantar lesions beneath the second, third, and/or fourth metatarsal heads.

Remember, the degree of metatarsus adductus can influence their position and such things as: patient activity, weight, condition of the skin, circulation, and believe it or not, shoe type can influence onset and degree of severity.

Common Plantar Lesions and Their Surgical Approach

There are some 38 different combinations of plantar lesions which can occur on the forefoot. Obviously, understanding biomechanical principles, recognizing which of them to consider, and being capable of applying these implications becomes paramount when deciding the surgical approach or the choice of procedure:

Solitary Second Metatarsal Head Lesions

A. Determine if there is a so-called plantar flexed second metatarsal by palpating the plantar plane of the metatarsal heads with the subtalar joint and midtarsal joint maintained in a neutral position. If the remaining four metatarsal heads (first, third, fourth, and fifth) can be visualized or determined to lie on the same plane while being maximally dorsi-flexed and this plane is located higher than that of the second metatarsal head in its maximum dorsiflexion, you may consider directing your surgical approach only to the involved second metatarsal.

B. Determine if there is hypermobility or subluxation of the first ray by moving it through its extremes of sagittal plane motion. If this range of motion is oriented above the level of the other metatarsal ranges of motion and action of the peroneus longus is weak, an assumption of first metatarsal hypermobility and/or subluxation can be made. If the remaining lesser metatarsals (second, third, fourth, and fifth) are determined to lie on the same plane and appear stable, surgical consideration should be directed towards the *first* metatarsal. Consider a closing plantar wedge osteotomy of the base of the first metatarsal so as to position the metatarsal head more plantarly but achieving it by a "bend in the bone." An opening wedge osteotomy of the dorsum of the base of the first metatarsal will achieve the same result and if bunion removal is carried out at the same time, a bony wedge can be fashioned from the exostosis. The opening wedge can also be maintained by a staple.

Functional control by orthotics, as soon post-operatively as possible, should eliminate the actual second metatarsal head lesion.

C. Determine if perhaps the second metatarsal head lesion represents a clinical manifestation of a so-called "functional" forefoot varus. On measurement from the first to the fifth metatarsal head, there is a varus reading but on measurement from the second to the fifth metatarsal head, there is a valgus reading with the third and fourth metatarsal heads lying on this valgus plane. If such a condition exists, one will probably see at least dispersive callous extending under the lateral metatarsal heads and if surgical intervention is directed only toward the second metatarsal, one can anticipate the so-called "transfer" lesions to appear beneath the third metatarsal head and subsequently the fourth metatarsal head. This general type of biomechanical abnormality has proved troublesome and one should not hesitate to surgically expand the metatarsal involvement by performing dorsal wedge osteotomies or extension osteoarthrotomies on both the second and third or the second, third, and fourth metatarsal bases.

On occasion, one might also consider including a first metatarsal plantar-flexory osteotomy with the second, third, and fourth dorsi-flexory procedures.

Solitary Third Metatarsal Head Lesions:

A. As with the second metatarsal head lesion, determine the presence of a true plantar-flexed third ray.

B. Determine if the etiologic factor might be strictly *closed*-chain pronation wherein there would be an affect on the medial three rays because of the adduction and plantar-flexion of the anterior articular facet of the head of the talus. You would have the navicular rotated on the frontal plane with the first ray on a higher plane and the articulation with the third ray on a lower plane (more or less the first and third pivoting about the middle or second cuneiform) and resulting in an overall positioning of the third metatarsal more toward the plantar surface of the foot.

Solitary Fourth Metatarsal Head Lesions

A. The fourth metatarsal, as I have mentioned earlier, must be treated with more attention because of the basal joint axis. The true plantar flexed fourth metatarsal requires a greater dorsi-flexory range of motion than the second metatarsal requires to elevate their metatarsal heads an equal amount.

B. Determine the presence of a plantar positioned fourth metatarsal by considering both closed and open chain pronation. In this situation, the calcaneus everts relative to the talus. The cuboid articulates with the calcaneus and will be everted also. The fourth and fifth metatarsal bases articulate with the cuboid and so, therefore, the axis of the fourth metatarsal base will move to a more parallel relationship with the sagittal plane and will thus result in the metatarsal being, overall, positioned more toward the weight-bearing surface. This must be correlated with all of the other things which are taking place and to which I have previously referred.

C. Apparently, because the fourth undergoes the least amount of movement during weight-bearing (stance and gait), we can tolerate some instability of the fourth metatarsophalangeal joint. Therefore, plantar condylectomy of this particular bone remains in the armamentarium and can be used with success at times.

Conclusion

In closing, I wish to reemphasize that the clinical plantar lesion may not be located directly beneath the metatarsal head that is producing the abnormal stresses because of the tri-plane motion taking place. Frequently, the callous and its corresponding metatarsal head are located oblique from each other. That is, the callous is located distal and lateral to its corresponding metatarsal head. This is especially true of the second and third.

I have not found it dependable to trust post-operative orthotic control to cover or substitute for inadequate and incomplete pre-surgical evaluation.

Summary

The understanding of both normal and abnormal biomechanics and its relationship to foot surgery is very important.

This importance is illustrated by a review of how a particular biomechanical abnormality influences a commonly operated clinical entity.

This clinical entity, associated with pain and disability in the foot, is the integumentary lesion on the plantar of the forefoot. The fixed osseous deformity — forefoot varus — is often found to be a predisposing cause of the plantar lesion beneath the internal lesser metatarsal heads.

A great variety of surgical procedures have been suggested in the treatment of these plantar lesions and, apparently, in podiatry, the most frequently used procedures involve the metatarsophalangeal joint.

When known biomechanical principles applicable to the internal lesser metatarsophalangeal joints are considered, a more logical, less destructive, and possibly more successful surgical approach is suggested.

Biomechanical Implications of Foot Surgery

Tilden H. Sokoloff

Biomechanical implications of foot surgery has become a popularly coined phrase within the past several years. Biomechanics is the science which deals with the relationship of structure and function. Surgery always deals with the relationship of structure and function, but when one begins to think of the biomechanical implications of a specific surgical technique, he views the technique a lot differently than just the skin opening, a bony resection and a skin closure. The thought processes which lead one to choose one technique over another should be based upon sound biomechanical principles which will help give a favorable prognosis as to the long-range success of the surgical technique employed.

We shall attempt to discuss the salient biomechanical relationships as they should be evaluated on every patient for whatever surgical procedure is contemplated. We will then proceed to go over a specific surgical procedure as an example of how biohemchanics influences surgery at a very relevant level.

When we say broad mechanical features or biomechanical features as affecting foot function, we are basically evaluating the structural abnormalities as related to the foot-leg relationship. We are basically evaluating the soft tissue abnormalities as related to the foot-leg relationship and we are evaluating how the patient compensates for whatever structural or soft tissue abnormalitiy is present. The greatest surgical technique could be performed on a patient who has an uncompensated type of deformity with improper evaluation, good surgical technique and poor postoperative management; naturally, the surgical procedure is destined to fail. Surgery should be looked at as a tripod stand of a camera. There are basically three legs to it: one is proper pre-operative evaluation, two is proper surgical technique, and three, and probably most important, is post-operative follow-up. Proper postoperative follow-up does not begin or end with the making or construction of an arch support. This is no longer adequate to insure the post-operative management of our patients. We will discuss this further later in the paper.

Tilden H. Sokoloff, D.P.M., *Director of Podiatric Surgery, California College of Podiatric Medicine, San Francisco, Calif.*

The patient who is being evaluated for surgical correction of a deformity, such as a plantarflexed first ray, hallux valgus, digital deformity, calcaneal heel pain problems, or any surgical procedure we perform should be evaluated through a simple type examination technique. It does not require the cumbersome measurement of joints; it does not require sophisticated equipment; but it does require a mental picture of what you hope to accomplish with the deformity that presents itself. The first portion of the examination should really deal with a basic review of the lower extremity as a whole, the internal and external rotation: are they equal or are they not equal? Two: the range of motion at the knee joint. Three: the range of motion at the ankle joint – Is there a limitation of ankle joint motion, is the limitation lessened when the knee is flexed indicating a possible gastrocnemius equinus deformity? Muscle power should be basically evaluated at the hip, knee and ankle joint to see whether there is a relative inadequacy of motion noted in any one specific muscle group. We do not have to get down to individual muscle testing but basically groups. Are they balanced? Is there enough motion to allow it to compensate for another muscle group, such as the anterior crural group versus the posterior crural group? We then basically want to evaluate subtalar joint motion and want to recognize whether or not there are any varus or valgus abnormalities of the subtalar joint. Are there any coalitions in the subtalar joint? Are there any bars present? We will compare this information with what we know about the midtarsal joint. Are there any varus or valgus rotations? Are there any plantarflexions noted in the lesser metatarsals? Is the first ray hypermobile? Is the first ray plantarflexed? This is information that can be obtained by just training your eye to visualize an entire extremity. It takes minutes without going into a sophisticated examination or into a detailed mechanical work-up on every patient. The surgeon should train himself to basically isolate deformities which will have a direct bearing on the surgical procedure that he is contemplating, so that he can adequately judge whether or not the placement of a joint in one position will maintain itself that way post-operatively. He wants to avoid the five and ten year follow-up that comes back to the office and says, "Doctor, why is my bunion back?" or "Doctor, why do I have a plantar callous again?" or "Doctor, why does the joint hurt?"

After this clinical evaluation, the best indication of foot function is to watch the patient walk, which is probably one of the most important parts of pre-operative evaluation. Gait observation is just one technique of training the clinician's eye to look for certain important components of the gait cycle. Gait is divided into two basic sections which we are all familiar with: 1) the swing phase and 2) the stance phase. The swing phase being that phase in which the limb is really not in contact with the ground and the stance phase being that portion of the gait cycle where the foot is in contact with the ground. In the stance phase, the first thing you are looking at as the patient is ambulating is basically the contact phase or the heel contact. This is approximately 25% of stance phase of gait. As you are watching heel contact, you are preparing yourself to look at the mid stance portion of gait which takes about 40% of the total time. And then you are watching for the propulsive phase of gait to see whether it is a propulsive gait or an apropulsive gait. The patient may not propel at all. The patient may have a very early heel off or be a toe walker. The patient may just roll off the side and externally rotate the whole limb and just not propel at all. These are the things that the eye has to pick up and these are the things that you want to know about this particular patient. The changes in the subtalar joint that you can train yourself to watch for, now that you have looked at the gross components of gait, are the position of heel to ground when it strikes, whether or not the subtalar joint goes through its pronatory range of motion and if it does, is the patient maximumly pronated in mid stance or not. These are things that you want to note. Does the patient assume the normal variations of motion from a neutral or slightly supinated position at heel contact to a pronated position on or before mid stance to a rather neutral position at mid stance and then to a supinated position for propulsion?

After you have gone through this examination which basically should take a very short period of time to gather some of the salient features, it is then a matter of "Well, what does it all mean?" Basically, now that you have obtained certain mechanical information, you can decide whether a patient has normal structure and function, or abnormal structure and function. Obviously, if there is a deformity present, there is some etiology present — for instance, the plantar keratoma. You have gone through the entire examination as we just discussed. You have evaluated the fact that the patient's subtalar joint is slightly in varus, that the midtarsal joint has a slightly varus deformity. Knowing some of the biomechanical implications of the presenting deformities, you will know that the patient with a subtalar deformity will pronate to get that heel fixed on the ground. Having a forefoot varus deformity, hypermobility of the first ray or an equinus deformity, will give you a pronatory tendency or a tendency to pronate through the gait cycle. If you have established this fact, and the patient has plantar lesions and you want to act upon this lesion surgically, you have decided that because of this pronation, there is a shearing force on the bottom of the foot. The foot is just going through an abnormal range of motion. So consequently, with this pronation, a loosening up of the midtarsal joint occurs, and will cause a hypermobility of the midtarsal joint; consequently you are going to get a shearing force across the bottom of the foot and you are going to develop lesions. Theoretically, if you control the foot, whatever the etiology is again and you controlled it with an orthotic, you should be able to get rid of the plantar lesion. But let's say clinically you have ascertained that the second and third metatarsal is plantarflexed. This is very hard to do except through an axial view on x-ray or through just good clinical evaluation where you place the foot in its neutral position and palpate the metatarsal heads to ascertain whether one metatarsal head is plantarflexed on another. So through a cursory examination, you have established the fact that the patient has a subtalar, midtarsal or deformity. You have established the fact that the patient has a plantarflexed second. You have also established the fact that the patient compensates by pronating through the gait cycle. Now you want to act upon this deformity. The difference between acting upon a deformity surgically with proper bio-mechanical evaluation versus just acting upon a deformity, when you change the biomechanics of the foot either with an orthotic or with attempting to change joint motion by way of surgery and then follow it up with orthotic therapy, is that you are basically dealing with a total structure and a total function; but when you operate on a plantar lesion and just resect the plantar condyles of a bone and just say, "Well, it was the plantar condyles that caused the callous and I have resected the plantar condyles and consequently the plantar callous will go away," you are really not changing or trying to change its function. Consequently, when you change the function and structure of a specific joint or a specific soft tissue structure, the implications of what you have done really are not felt until adequate post-operative follow-up occurs. When we start to talk in terms of biomechanical evaluation and not just use a fancy term which impresses people, we are basically talking about how to change the function of a joint, how to maintain it with proper post-operative follow-up, and more importantly, we understand the changes that are occurring in that joint due to surgery.

When we discuss the principles of proper orthopedic care or biomechanical care after surgery, we are basically discussing several broad principles. *One* is to eliminate the abnormal forces or structures. *Two* is to try to neutralize abnormal forces or structures. *Three* is to try to counteract these abnormal forces or structures by use of an external means or we want to protect or accommodate an area of symptomology. If you break this down in your mind and discuss the biomechanical follow-up of a surgical patient with one of these broad headings in mind, then the use of different modalities will play a bigger role in your practice, plus it will perform a specific function for you post-operatively. Now the prognosis of everything that you are doing really depends upon your ability to eliminate abnormal function and you guide this by eliminating the symptoms the patient is relating and by getting rid of certain signs that you clinically see. In other words, you do a hallux valgus deformity correction, the patient has a pronatory type problem, the patient pronates through gait, you put an external device in his shoe and you watch the patient ambulate and you still see him pronate and you still see the first metatarsal phalangeal joint going through some subluxatory changes; you know that your post-operative period is destined to fail. You know that the patient is going to get the deformity back only because you have not sufficiently maintained the position of this patient's foot so that this abnormal force can no longer pass through the entire foot. It is easy to slap plaster on a foot, send it out to the lab and have an orthotic made. It is hard to think about why and what you are doing and what you want to accomplish and be able to identify when you are not accomplishing it. That is the most important factor. When one takes a negative cast for an orthotic, try to keep the forefoot and rearfoot relationship in that cast so that you can counteract the forces in that foot with some mechanical means. For example: a post which will stop a specific area from going through an abnormal range of motion or a cast correction which will accomplish this on the positive cast or any method you wish to employ.

Post-operative x-rays should be employed regularly. When mechanical considerations have been employed for surgical correction, keep tabs on what is happening. When you perform a surgical procedure, you have months in which this joint is basically a mobile structure that you can put into various positions by either taping, casting, orthotics, bracing or any other method. The patients must understand that when surgery is undertaken for the correction of a major deformity, that it is not how fast we put them back in their fashionable shoes, because we get them back and they love us the first year or the second year, but five years later that toe is deformed again and they cannot understand why – "My doctor operated on me, he put me in the hospital and did a fine job, he told me I'd be back to work in four weeks, he had me back in shoes in four weeks and now all of a sudden, I have the same deformity back." It is because we kidded ourselves and we kidded the patient as to the overall management of the deformity.

The mechanical follow-up of these patients is the most important part of the whole procedure. We are getting ourselves involved in more major types of foot surgery. Podiatry has gone through an era where we have done as much destructive surgery as any other surgical specialty. We had a hammertoe, we opened the joint, we took the head of the proximal phalanx and we restored it back to the transverse plane. We reduced a hallux valgus by resecting the base of the proximal phalanx because the toe was so subluxed, we had no choice. Now we are getting into times where we are talking about reconstructive surgery. What can we do to restore the structures that are present at this time? This creates the most interesting and rewarding types of foot surgery that we can offer our patients and the medical profession. But to insure the proper technique and proper follow-up is the responsibility of the operating surgeon.

I hope that through this short discussion of some of the philosophies of biomechanical implications to foot surgery, we can better understand the need for better post-operative care. And then we will realize that the surgical technique is really the smallest portion of the total surgical care.

The Importance of the Physical Examination in Podiatric Treatment

The first and major function of a physician is to perform adequate history and physical examination. History taking is an art worthy of the doctor's personal attention. This history must be adequate and it must be accurate. The physical examination and history must be of sufficient amount so that the physician may form a tentative diagnosis. What I hate to see most of all is a physician who skips directly from the chief complaint to the laboratory diagnosis. This is the doctor who simply walks into the room to hear the patient's chief complaint of "My foot hurts" or "My back hurts". This doctor's response usually is "Let's get an x-ray." Very little clinical information is given to the radiologist who therefore cannot act as a consultant, and in truth has great difficulty in performing adequate service. The films are made. The physician views the films, and nine out of ten times, as you well know, the films are normal. Then the physician is left in a most difficult position because he has no idea of what ails the patient because he has relied upon a laboratory diagnostic measure. He has not listened to the patient and he has not examined him. He has not formulated a tentative diagnosis. The net result is that he very frequently finds himself in the position of saying, "I cannot do anything for you, let's just wait." It seems to me that this is precisely the wrong approach. The medical history is an extremely important part of any medical examination. The physician must listen to the patient, but he must not let the patient ramble on and on. As he is listening to the patient, the physician must formulate some idea as to the diagnosis and then insert questions to test that hypothesis. The questions will direct the patient and keep him from wandering into minute details that are of no importance. In addition, it will keep the physician's mind on the task which he faces.

It is important to listen to the patient, to obtain the chief complaint and to elaborate upon it. The chief complaint is not the patient's diagnosis. Very frequently the patient will give you his diagnosis. He may be right, and in this case the physician's task is easy. On the other hand, the patient may be wrong,

James S. Miles, M.D. *University of Colorado Medical Center, Denver, Colorado.*

and the physician's task is made much more complex. I hasten to add that this is a process which is quite familiar to us as physicians and to many other business and professional men. All of you have had the experience of taking your automobile into the garage to put it into the tender hands of a mechanic. Frequently you tell the mechanic that you want the carburetor tuned up or that you want the sparkplugs changed. The wise mechanic advises you that he is not interested in your desires but wants to know your chief complaint with regard to the automobile. He wants to know if the automobile has lost its pep, if it's gasoline mileage has decreased, or if there is a great deal of black smoke pouring out of the exhaust pipe. These latter items are symptoms of the disease of the automobile. You may well be correct that the carburetor or the sparkplugs are at fault, but you may also be wrong – and at great expense to you.

The case history as presented by the patient may be long and rambling, and this is the reason why many physicians try to avoid the taking of a history, or assign it to an office nurse or an associate. It is not necessary that you let the patient waste a great deal of time for you. Your time is valuable. You should not just sit there and listen to the patient's rambling account of what he thinks he has, or what he thinks is important. You must interrupt him from time to time in interest of accuracy and understanding. Words may well have a different meaning to you and the patient. These words cannot be accurately defined unless they are made objective. The word "pain" must be carefully discussed. Other inaccurate words must be qualified so that complete understanding is reached. For example, the patient may state that he has had his "pain" only a short time. To the physician this may mean a few days. To the patient, this may mean a few years. History taking is an active, vital conversation between the patient and the doctor. It must be directed by the physician so that it will be of benefit to all.

It is not my purpose here to enter into a discussion of interprofessional relationships. However, I am sure all of us realize that we violate professional ethics very, very frequently, either from ignorance, because of the lack of time, or because of the demands of the patient. In taking the history, the physician is most likely to determine if the patient is simply "shopping around" or "checking up" on his physician, or is sincerely interested in a professional consultation. Many times we have patients calling our Orthopedic Clinic simply asking for an appointment. My nurse, who handles these calls, is very adroit at getting from the callers the story of their previous medical care. Quite a few patients become irate at these questions. Very often they seek to humble my nurse by stating that they are going to pay for this visit, that they have a right to choose their own doctor, and that they do not have time for all of these questions. My nurse very calmly then tells the patients that we would like to give them the best possible consultation and in order to do this we must have all of the clinical information. Information cannot be supplied by the patient but should be supplied by the referring physician. I must hasten to add that in trying to maintain proper professional relationships and good medical ethics, we have cut down a great deal on the talk of malpractice suits and other such complications.

I frequently encounter another situation in which the taking of an adequate history helps me to keep the patient. So many times I find myself confronted with a confused or distressed patient, whose previous medical care has been perfectly adequate. I may myself wish to recommend exactly the same course of therapy which had previously been advised. If I were simply to advise such, the patient often becomes very irate, saying that "That's what everyone else has been advising me to do, but it simply hasn't worked." Or the patient may quietly leave – very disgusted with the medical profession. In the taking of a history in this situation, I ask the patient to give me more information regarding the supposedly ineffective treatment, and I can most often determine why the treatment has not succeeded. I may feel that the best treatment is a brace or a corset. In the taking of the history, I may hear that the patient has tried "dozens of corsets." I must then determine if the corsets have been used adequately. I have even found one unsuccessful and disgruntled brace wearer who had been wearing the brace upside down. Simply showing the man how to wear the brace not only resulted in a cure, but restored the patient's confidence in our profession. I have frequently found that the treatment advice has not been carried out by the patient. In many instances whatever medical therapy has been advised, has been accepted with a half-hearted or very uncooperative attitude. The prime example of this is an exercise program, both for range of motion, and for muscle strength. Patients very often are uncooperative in the active aspects of these exercises and are more than willing to leave the exercises to the passive efforts of a physical therapist. Confronted by a patient who angrily tells me that he has been advised to exercise in the past, I simply ask him to demonstrate the exercises for me and to show me the record of his exercise sessions while at home. Almost every time I can then point out to the patient the inadequacy of his efforts and stress to him that his getting well is a matter of his effort as well as that of the doctor or the therapist.

Next in the physical examination, I would urge that you organize yourself so that you can examine the patient properly and obtain all the meaningful information necessary. We teach the medical students to examine the extremities from the standpoint of tissue priorities. With regard to survival and function of an extremity, these tissues should be considered in the following order – vascular, skin, nerve, tendon, joint, bone, and muscle.

Let me simply illustrate how each of these tissues may be evaluated in an orderly and purposeful fashion. Injury or disease of any of these tissues may be productive of symptoms. In addition, the treatment of any problem may be complicated by associated, or non-related disease or injury. For example, the treatment of a closed metatarsal fracture is quite different from the treatment of an open metatarsal fracture which results from a crush injury with skin loss, nerve and tendon damage.

An adequate evaluation of the vascular supply of the extremity includes examination not only of the arterial, but also the venous and lymphatic supply. Swelling of the extremity and pigmentation of the skin may be an indication of postphlebitic change with inadequacy of venous return.

Most medical students are surprised that skin is placed at such a high degree of priority. However, it is quite obvious that before any tissues other than vascular can be repaired, one must plan for skin coverage. Not only should one look for evidence of injury of the skin, but also to the health of the skin and its appendages. The smooth, glistening skin with pigmentation is quite a different tissue from normal skin with it's normal subcutaneous tissue, normal hair, normal nail growth, normal sweat glands. The atrophic damaged skin will not tolerate swelling. Nor will it tolerate trauma, either accidental or surgical.

Nerve supply must be evaluated, both motor and sensory. An adequate knowledge of anatomy is necessary for a meaningful neurologic examination, and such examinations may become quite technical and involved.

Tendon function is of greater importance than muscle function, because obviously the tendon must glide through a normal range of excursion in order to have normal function. There are specialized areas where tendon function is of much greater importance than nerve function. This is particularly true on the flexor aspect of the hand and fingers. Again, to evaluate tendon function accurately, one must have knowledge of anatomy of the hand or the area involved. It is extremely important that one separate extrinsic muscle and tendon function from intrinsic muscle and tendon function, for example.

Joint function is next in importance because joint surfaces must be congruent in order for normal function to exist. One must be concerned not only with the articular cartilage and the actual joint contact, but also with the tissues which surround the joint and contribute to its function. I refer to the capsule, the ligaments, and in many areas, menisci and surrounding tendons. Joint ranges of motion must be recorded objectively. Any chart which simply records ankle joint motion as being "pretty good", toe motion as "not so bad" and knee joint motion as "unremarkable" is absolutely useless. The joint range of motion must be recorded in degrees in standard fashion so that subsequent examinations by the original physician or by other physicians may be similarly made and compared.

Bone is next in importance. I am often questioned by medical students as to my reason for placing my favorite tissue in such a low degree of priority. I do so because bone has such a remarkable capacity for repair. It is the one tissue of the body which repairs itself by replacing itself. Skin will do so in a very limited fashion but not as perfectly as bone. An evaluation of bone injury or disease must record exactly the point of maximal tenderness and the anatomic site must be accurately recorded.

Last in importance is muscle, last only because muscle function may be substituted. The patient may well use substitute muscles or the surgeon may transfer muscles and tendons in order to restore or replace function.

One may well question the reason for doing so careful a history and physical examination. I can only give you my firm belief that this is fundamental to the establishment of a working diagnosis and a final diagnosis. It is often so extremely important from a medical-legal standpoint and probably will become more important from a governmental standpoint, as the government takes more and more control of medical practice. Lastly, this is the primary method of establishing good doctor-patient relationships which are so important to patient care and for our status as professional men.

VI. Evaluation of Soft Tissue Injuries of the Foot and Ankle

Panel Discussion

Moderator: George S. Gill

Panelists: Milton Fulp, Joseph Doller,
C. Robert Starks

DR. FULP: I'd like to confine my dissertation to a few areas — primarily, ankle joint injuries. While I was in high school playing football, I began suffering a tremendous amount of ankle sprains and they were subsequently diagnosed (characteristically) as negative for fracture. The powers-that-be wrapped the injury in an Ace bandage and sent me home. Since this period of time, I have also suffered a torn ligament in the knee and a severe fracture of the upper right arm. Both the latter healed fine, but unfortunately I still have ankle-joint problems. I was virtually a cripple while I was in podiatry school and ended up having to have a Watson Jones procedure and being placed in and out of the cast for over six months. I think that the old adage of the sprained ankle being often much worse than a broken ankle is very true, but primarily because of one reason only; when any of us sees a fractured ankle joint, we automatically cast it, of course. As long as the osseous structure heals, the ligamentous structure generally heals also. Where we get into real trouble, however, is when we see ankle joint injuries with no fracture. Generally, no stress view or no arthrogram is taken, and there is really no way for us to assess just how much ligamentous instability has occurred. So — all in all — we tend to treat these occurrences rather lightly. I think that both the podiatric profession and that of orthopedic surgeons — or, indeed, any persons who deal with joints as a specialty — have to be held accountable for a higher level of care than that generally accepted in the medical profession.

It was assumed before arthrographic examination was possible that a tear in the distal tibial fibular ligament virtually never occurs without a concomitant

George S. Gill, D.P.M., *Denver, Colorado;* Milton Fulp, D.P.M., *Doctors Hospital, Tucker, Georgia;* Joseph Doller, D.P.M., *Assistant Director, Athletics, Florida Institute of Technology, Melbourne, Florida;* C. Robert Starks, Sr., D.O., *President, Colorado Board of Medical Examiners, Denver, Colorado.*

tear in the deltoid ligament. The common lateral collateral injury is one that every one of us sees many times. I think we have to diagnose this injury in a couple of ways. First, there is the clinical symptom, tenderness on palpation, in the area of the lateral collateral ligament which, as we remember, consists of three bands: the anterior and posterior talofibular and the fibular calcaneal ligament being the central band. Also (if we remember our anatomy) we realize that the ankle joint tends to widen and narrow on dorsiflexion or plantarflexion so this injury normally occurs in a plantar flexed or neutral attitude, with generally the first ligament torn being the anterior part of the lateral collateral ligament. I think that this injury can be adequately diagnosed on stress views. Often it is necessary to do a common peroneal block as the everters go into a protective spasm and sometimes this is somewhat misleading and we may not get a true talar tilt in the mortise. Many articles discuss the number of degrees, etc. I think it is evident when you get a talar tilt and compare it with the other extremity, that you do have pathology.

Briefly, the arthrogram is done with a radiopaque iodine dye, either Hypaque or Conray, a 50% solution which is diluted 50% with 1% plain Xylocaine. The dye is introduced into the medial aspect of the joint — as most of our injuries, of course, are lateral ones. In the normal ankle joint the synovia and the ligamentous structures are contiguous. Therefore, we form a pouch that holds the contrast media. In an eversion or inversion sprain the ligaments are torn, the synovium is torn, and the dye can extravasate into the soft tissues of the leg. I refer you to an excellent article in the December, 1970 issue of *Journal of Bone and Joint Surgery* written by Dr. Gordon, an orthopedist from San Francisco, who did most of the original work on arthrograms in this country.

There is no substitute for an arthrogram in a case where there is suspicion of the widening of the ankle joint mortise, the dye leaking out as a confirmatory sign. Obviously, a severe talar tilt tells you the story. It is probably of no additional value to do an arthrogram in this instance; however, in a case, where you suspect a rupture of the distal tibifibular ligament, this then is confirmatory and I think extremely helpful.

The treatment for widening of the mortise is to put a transverse screw across the mortise to tighten up the mortise. The patient is casted for six weeks and the screw then removed. Please remember that this is a joint that we are dealing with; in which there is motion. The screw should not remain in the joint since, if it should break, it can't very easily be removed.

I know that we are confining ourselves to soft-tissue injuries. Of course, with a fracture there is going to be severe capsular damage. You can expect to see a mass of leakage of the contrast media in an injury of this magnitude.

The next area I would like to discuss is the question of the digital crush injuries that every one of us sees in our offices very often involving young, healthy patients. We notice a tremendous amount of venous engorgement, probably due to venous thrombosis, both superficial and deep. I think that the mechanism of action in the gangrenous toes that we too often see following severe crush injuries, is probably due more to venous engorgement than to arterial insufficiency. I find something useful: take 10 mg of Depo Heparin and dissolve it in low-molecular weight Dextran 40, and inject it into the arterial or venous tree of the lower extremity as close to the injured digit as you can, or inject it *directly* into the affected digit. It seems to help in rechannelling the vascular tree in the digit and thus prevent venous engorgement.

Another topic I wish to go into is the Achilles tendon rupture. With the advent of more tendo-Achilles lengthenings in our profession, I think that we are going to be faced more often with postoperative rupture of the tendo-Achilles. I have seen a couple of them myself in the two years that I have been at Doctors' Hospital and both resulted from a careless patient *stepping* off a curb too vigorously — with resultant severe pain and complete rupture of the ligament. Of course, patients come in to see you. They have a difficult time walking. Indeed, they may not be able to walk at all. They are in acute pain, so you lie them down prone, the feet protruding from the end of the examining table, and you do a Simmons test. This means squeezing the calf muscle, which should cause movement at the ankle joint. With complete rupture of the tendo Achilles, this won't occur. Therapy depends upon what sort of ligamentous tissue you find when you get in there. You may discover that you can sew it back together although you may need primarily to use the plantaris or one of the brevis tendons as a graft. I think this is something of which we all need to be cognizant and when we undertake to do a surgical procedure, we must also accept responsibility if our work goes somewhat awry.

I would also like to mention the tremendous increase in the number of Gram negative infections we see these days in the hospital. Staph aureus, or the "Golden Killer" of the hospital, seems to be pretty much under control. Instead, we are now identifying infections such as proteus, pseudomonas, and E. coli. The tendo-Achilles procedure is an excellent area in which to get one of these and they are absolutely devastating! We had one in a 7-8 year old white male patient, a very healthy boy. We did his tendo-Achilles lengthenings bilaterally with the typical two-skin incisions and slide procedure. He became infected unilaterally. He had a temperature of 105; the culture and sensitivity came back a Gram negative organism. He was sensitive only to Chloromycetin and Carbinocillin with which you may not be familiar. This is a new penicillin analog marketed under two names: Cylopen, Pyoren. It is given in massive doses of up to 20-25 grams per day. The drug companies are constantly pleading for all physicians to save this type of medication for Gram negative infections that don't respond to anything else. I gave this patient Betadine injections around the tendon to force the material out. He responded to the Cylopen. We gave it to him intravenously initially, and then intramuscularly. We kept him in an extra week. Under local anesthesia, we then took him back to the operating room, debrided and closed the skin injuries, and he has done very well since. I submit these two complications to you today for your consideration, because — sooner or later — as we do more and more of this sort of surgery, all of us are going to be faced with these kinds of complications.

DR. DOLLER: I would like to bring to your attention for discussion three soft tissue problems. One is called the tarsal tunnel syndrome, sometimes called tibial nerve entrapment, a difficult syndrome to treat. Some of us are wondering if the symptoms presented really indicate a tarsal tunnel syndrome or tibial nerve entrapment. The symptoms of the syndrome are usually related to an old ankle sprain type of injury. Although at the time the injury was assumed to be on the lateral side of the ankle, the medial side of the ankle has remained painful. Perhaps pain on the medial side is first realized when you exert some force against this area. One of the symptoms that is associated with the tarsal tunnel syndrome is a burning sensation. This symptom we have relieved in about 10 cases with aspiration of 3-5 cc of fluid and injection of an anesthetizing agent.

The anatomy of the area consists of the sulcus on the dorsum of the calcaneus and the corresponding sulcus on the plantar side of the body of the talus which is filled with the interosseus talocalcaneal ligament. It is from this sulcus that we have aspirated fluid, injected anesthesia, and the pain has disappeared. We are considering then if it is accumulation of fluid within the confines of the tunnel pressing against the interosseous membranes of the talocalcaneal ligament which is causing the symptoms rather than a nerve entrapment problem.

The second problem that I would like to mention for your consideration is the famous Morton's neuroma and nerve entrapment of the interdigital areas. I am not going to review the well-known signs and symptoms. I would like you to consider how many times the surgeon has told you that he operated for a Morton's neuroma but found only normal nerve fibers. We are wondering if this is always a true nerve entrapment or a mild fasciitis of the lumbricales muscles in an area usually associated with Morton's neuroma syndrome. One of our diagnostic methods to differentiate muscle from nerve involvement is to inject anesthesia along with a cortisone type preparation in the area; if the syndrome disappears we believe that it was a soft tissue envolvement rather than a nerve entrapment.

Another problem which I would like to mention is the heel spur syndrome. The differential diagnoses which might be considered are: (a) plantar calcaneal nerve entrapment; (b) heel spur syndrome associated with electrolyte imbalance occurring in persons who are taking diuretics and who are often overweight. Orthopods usually refer to this syndrome as plantar fasciitis. How much of the plantar fascia actually involved with the presenting heel spur syndrome is a matter of clinical judgment. (c) Malalignment of the calcaneus, with or without relationship to a subtalar alignment, must be considered; (d) arthritic involvement; and (e) gout-associated syndrome.

MODERATOR: Dr. Fulp, please give diagnostic points and x-ray positioning for rupture and separation of the lateral talocalcaneal ligament, and please give percentage of solutions used for arthrograms.

DR. FULP: A clinical examination of an ankle sprain is the first procedure. Often, with palpation over the lateral collateral ligaments and with forcible inversion, you can feel the talus and it slips out of the mortise and down away from the fibula. Sometimes there is a palpable groove. If you are careful, this can be carried out without anesthetizing the patient.

Sometime anterior-posterior, oblique, and lateral x-ray views will rule out a fracture. For stress views, turn the foot so that the malleoli parallel the film and then forcibly invert the foot. It may or may not be necessary to do a peroneal block. Some men won't do a stress view unless the patient is under general anesthesia because of the muscular spasm. At that time, if they find a tremendous amount of talar instability, they do a primary repair of the ligaments.

Concerning the dilutions and solutions of the contrast media, there are two that I have used. One of them is "Hypaque;" the other is "Conray". Both are iodine derivatives, so they are contraindicated in persons with iodine sensitivity. They come in 50% concentrations which we dilute 50% with plain 1% Xylocaine. I believe that this accomplishes two purposes: (1) the chances of a reaction are reduced because the strength of the medication is reduced; and (2) the Xylocaine has a therapeutic effect and the patient feels better.

The contrast media and the Xylocaine are mixed together in a large 10-12 cc syringe and set aside. Then, after a good Betadine or pHisohex preparation, using very careful aseptic technique, the ankle joint is entered medially with a small needle and a skin wheal is made. Then with a large 1½" 21 gauge needle, you can go into the ankle joint with a 2 cc syringe full of 0.5% Xylocaine. You then detach the syringe and you will get a small amount of sanguinous-stained joint fluid coming back through the needle. You then attach the larger syringe and gently fill up the ankle cavity with the diagnostic solution (contrast media and Xylocaine). The patient will tell you when he has had enough. He will begin to feel pressure on the lateral side. When the patient says, "Stop!" add one more cc and then put a little negative pressure on the syringe and withdraw it quickly. If you don't put negative pressure on the syringe you will leave an iodine track in the tissue as you withdraw the needle.

DR. STARKS: I would like to comment on some soft tissue injuries regarding certain treatments and judgments. After a fracture or a sprain, there is always a problem in after care of the soft tissue injury. I think that often we are too anxious to get the individuals up and around right away. A patient with an ordinary sprain (not a lateral collateral ligament rupture) may give us more trouble in soft tissue injury by immediately getting him on his feet. The first 48 hours after a sprain is the most important time to keep the foot elevated; if you have ever seen a frozen foot from a sprain this is easily realized. I certainly disagree with injecting a local anesthetic into a ligament or into a sprained area with the idea of getting the person back on his feet, or into athletic contests immediately. Often we have more trouble with soft tissue injury than with a fracture, especially with continued swelling. I believe that if we can protect the foot with elevation, with ice and rest for the first few days after a sprain, we have done more for the patient than by getting him up and about regardless of whether a cast was applied or not. Soft tissue injuries deserve respect.

Another question which has been brought up is: How often do you open up these cases? The less operational procedures that are done on the foot, the better off you are. We don't open up every lateral collateral ligament rupture. These will heal if given proper treatment. This morning we saw a tilting of the astragalus. The main feature in managing this case was to obtain a direct line down through the tibia through the talus so that proper weight-bearing is obtained. I attended a clinic in California in which 60 cases of fracture of the medial and lateral malleolus were presented. The main feature in their management, again, was obtaining proper weight-bearing. I must emphasize that nature does a lot of healing of soft tissues when the tissue is given a chance to rest.

Another comment that I would like to make is in reference to heel spurs. Bursitis was not mentioned as a factor to be considered. We should remember that nature protects attachment to the os calcis by the plantar fascia by production of a bursitis. The injection of procaine or Xylocaine with some Hydeltra, will take care of many of them. You are going to have many failures if you don't change the shoes or the weight-bearing with the shoes and change the os calcis direction by the shoes. Generally, these people have an external rotation of the os calcis and that puts a tension on the fascia that attaches to the os calcis. The heels must be raised and the shoe fit changed to get some relief.

MODERATOR: We have a few questions directed to Dr. Fulp.

DR. FULP: The first question is: "Why should you use heparin with Dextran for treatment of venous engorgement when Dextran is a plasma expander?" The venous engorgement is the result of venous thrombosis and low molecular weight Dextran, or Dextran 40, seems to coat the erythrocytes with some sort of electrostatic charge which causes them to repel each other and seems to prevent palisading, clumping, and some of the typical clotting problems that we have.

The second question asks: "What are the parameters of primary surgical intervention in soft tissue injuries of the ankle, particularly involving the medial-collateral, the lateral-collateral, and inferior talofibular?" Let us begin with the last, the inferior talofibular. If you have a widening of the ankle mortise, you have one of two choices: (1) you may put a screw across the mortise of the ankle; or (2) you may put it in a cast and use firm manual compression. With the lateral-collateral or medial-collateral tear you also have two choices: (1) you may cast it for 6-8 weeks; or (2) do a primary repair. I don't have much experience with a torn deltoid ligament; it is an unfrequent injury. However, I do know that the medial-collateral ligament, rather than a tear, more frequently evulses bone and you are almost dealing with a fracture.

The next question is: "Do you copiously irrigate the rima with antibiotic solutions at the time of primary treatment?" The answer is: "Yes."

The next question asks me to outline a treatment regimen for the common ankle sprain. First, you have the responsibility of differentiating between a partial tear and a complete rupture. A partial tear can be treated with ice immediately and later heat, rest, and immobilization; but when a complete lateral collateral tear exists, there are differences of opinion. Many suggest primary repair, and others suggest that plaster immobilization is quite adequate. This is a matter of personal preference, although the diagnosis of a partial tear or complete rupture is the physician's responsibility.

The last question is, "Please explain the best approach for introducing dye into the ankle?" You can locate the sulcus between the extensor hallucis longus and the anterior tibial tendon and introduce the dye at this point under good aseptic technique. The ankle mortise can be located by palpation. You may have to feel and probe around a bit but be patient, and because local anesthesia is successful, you won't hurt the patient at all.

DR. STARKS: The next question: "What is your advice for follow-up treatment of ankle injuries in the young athlete?" "Also, in one in which there are recurrent problems?"

Our procedure is this. After taking x-rays and making tests which have already been suggested here, we determine how severe the injury is. If there is marked swelling, we put the patient to bed with elevation, compression and ice packs. The compression is done with the use of webril and elastoplast. This is continued for forty-eight hours when maximum swelling occurs. We then put the patient on crutches and graduated weight-bearing is allowed.

It is difficult to keep young kids off their feet. We follow-up this immediate treatment with stirrup strapping so that we will prevent excessive lateral medial movement. Graduated weight-bearing is allowed. Also, coaches or trainers are instructed to use the stirrup strapping whenever the boy participates in athletics.

I want to comment also on the use of various drugs which are supposed to diminish the swelling. Someone has well said that you can do a lot of things to defeat nature and also a lot of things to help nature. I think however, we sometimes go overboard and incline to the former. For example, we get a swollen ankle and are sure we should give the patient something to bring it down. The main thing is to realize just what we do; we do hinder nature many times and this is one of those times! So we don't inject swollen ankles with any type of hyaluronidase for that very reason. We think it is more important to stay on the fundamental principles of elevation, compression and ice. This is 98% of the therapy as far as I am concerned. We no longer use any type of injections into the swelling, nor do we use any medication by mouth for the swelling.

DR. DOLLER: I would like to interject a thought in regard to the management of sprained ankles. There are those among us who are hospital-oriented, and those who are office-oriented. Each orientation contributes to the way in which we might manage a particular condition. Certainly all the facilities found in a hospital or emergency clinic are not found in the average office.

There are other things, too, to be considered: (1) how old is the patient; is he a youngster, a teenager, a young adult, or an older adult; (2) in an x-ray picture, are you looking at an old broken-off piece of an arthritic osseous nodule that has been laying there for 15 years or are you looking at a new fracture? In treating an acute ankle sprain and you are sure you are not dealing with a fracture or dislocation, the only treatment called for is elevation, ice, and compression — if these three things are not done within the first 12-24 hours the patient is going to have a long period of convalescence whatever treatment is subsequently carried out.

I might add at this point that I was involved in the early use by injection of hyaluronidase enzyme. I found no particular value for this chemical when we used it in prime healthy athletic individuals 20-35 years of age. Rest, elevation and compression remain the principal therapeutic modalities; however, we also use some type of cold pack. I would like to pass on to you a therapeutic pearl mentioned on another panel. A 4" Ace bandage is saturated with water and placed in the freezing compartment of a refrigerator for use as needed. It stays there indefinitely until the first acute problem shows up when the ice pack is used to compress the foot. In conjunction with this, rather than using the simple tensor bandage with ice applied by some other means, cotton batting or a combination of roll batting and sponge compression or urethane mold is used. The patient is sent home on crutches and is told to keep off his feet and return to the office the next day for followup.

DR. STARKS: I have been asked the following question: "What is your opinion about the possibility of a cuboid lesion and subluxation being overlooked in an ankle sprain, and can this be treated by manipulation?" I would say that this and the rotation of the os calcis are the common conditions overlooked. The continuation of difficulties in the foot and ankle may be entirely due to these lesions.

VII. Treatment of Clubfoot— Conservative vs. Surgical

Treatment of Clubfoot — Conservative vs. Surgical

Thomas E. Sgarlato

My subject today is limited to a discussion of the levels of deformity and the variations that can be present at each level. We do not claim to be experts in therapy for foot deformities. We generally are limited to providing therapy to approximately a half dozen patients each year. Most patients with a congenital club foot deformity are screened at birth, thus we tend only to see those that are mismanaged or overlooked. Clinically, there appears to be four main levels of deformity present, (1) the ankle joint, (2) the talocalcaneal joint, (3) the midtarsal joint which has two segments, the talonavicular and calcaneal cuboid segment and (4) Lisfranc joint. The latter is metatarsal cuneiforms and metatarsal cuboidal joints. Here we have the diagram of the foot structure with clear demonstration of the various levels. At each level where there is a potential deformity there are two possible types which can be present, individually or collectively. The first is the structural type whereby the shape of bone is altered in a manner to effect joint position. The second is a positional type. This would be where the shape of the osseous structure is essentially normal initially; however, because of a mal joint position, the osseous structure eventually becomes secondarily deformed. The positional deformity is related to soft tissue maintenance which is a contractural state of muscles and/or anomalous tendons with ligamentous anomalies and other periarticular structures potentially participating. Of the two types of deformities, therapeutically positional deformities are the easiest to correct as one needs to only change the position of one part to another around the joint, whereas structural deformities are more difficult to correct because one must change the shape of the osseous structure to achieve full correction. This I believe accounts for the large amount of lack of definition of the deformity and inconsistency in providing therapy for clubfoot

Thomas E. Sgarlato, D.P.M., *Director of Biomechanics Department and Professor of Surgery, California College of Podiatric Medicine, California Podiatry Hospital and Outpatient Department, San Francisco, Calif.*

deformities in past literature. And that is the lack of differentiating structural and positional deformities at each level.

The first level we will discuss will be the Lisfranc joint. The Lisfranc joint deformity where a metatarsus adductus deformity of the foot is at the metatarsal cuneiform and metatarsal cuboidal joint.

(Figure 1). Here we see a Lisfranc joint adductus deformity very graphically in a child who is approximately 6-months-old.

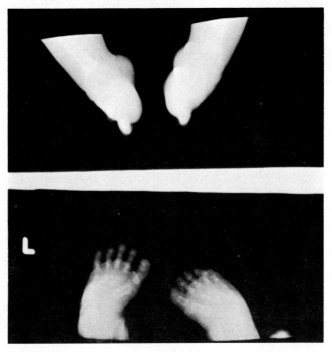

Figure 1.

This deformity can be assessed by measuring the relationship of the lesser tarsus to the metatarsals using the second metatarsal as a criteria. Any angulation above approximately 30 degrees would be considered a deformity.

The next level that we see is a deformity at the midtarsal or choparts joint. This a combination of the talonavicular and calcaneal cuboid joint. If one were to draw a solid line bisecting the os calcis one would find that the center of the ossified portion of the cuboid in an infant should fall right directly on that line. If the center of the ossified portion of the cuboid is medial to that line, then there is a calcaneal cuboid adduction or supinatory deformity. The talonavicular joint deformity can only be visualized by interpretation as the navicular is not ossified at an early age. However, when the talus is markedly superimposed on the os calcis the only space available for the navicular to ossify or be present in its cartilagenous state is medial. This level of the deformity is related to a contractural state of the posterior tibial muscle, if muscle is involved. Whereas the Lisfranc joint deformity would be related to a contractural state of the abductor hallucis muscle.

(Figure 2). Here is the radiograph of a choparts joint and Lisfranc joint deformity in a four-year-old child.

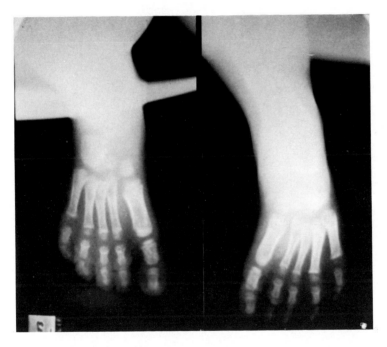

Figure 2.

(Figure 3). On a lateral view we can see the manifestation of the first ray apparatus including the mevicular on the talus along with the dorsiflexion of metatarsals five and four on the cuboid in the direction of a rocker bottom. This demonstrates the changes at the midtarsal joint level in planes other than the transverse plane, specifically the frontal plane and sagittal plane showing a relative valgus or varus of the forepart of the foot to the rearfoot and abnormal dorsiflexion of the forefoot on the rearfoot.

(Figure 4). Here is another radiograph of the first ray plantarflexed on the talus and the fifth and fourth metatarsals dorsiflexed on the cuboid, from the lateral radiograph.

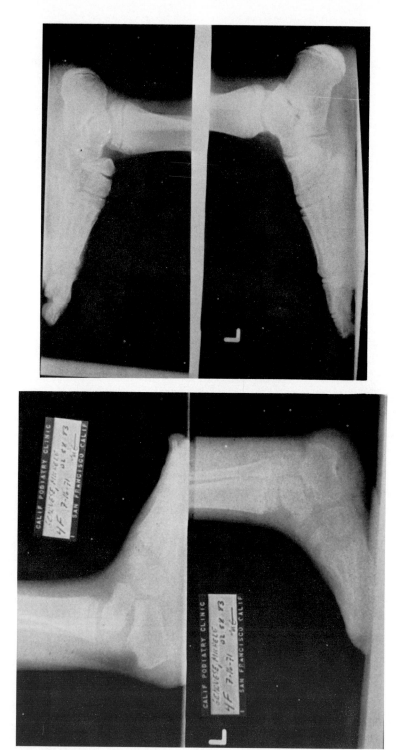

Figure 4.

Figure 3.

The next level we will discuss will be the talocalcaneal joint. There are two potential deformities present at this joint: (1) structural being the shape of the os calcis with the varus twist and/or the shape of the talus; (2) positional being the maximum supinatory position around the talocalcaneal joint.

(Figure 5). Our illustration here demonstrates a normal talocalcaneal range of excursion. Number 1, being a full supinatory position. Number 3, being a full pronatory position. If the varus deformity of the talocalcaneal joint is positional,

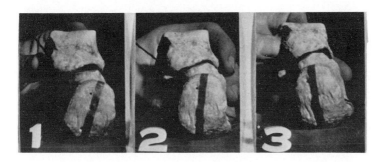

Figure 5.

then the structures would look as they do in Number 1. The foot would simply be fully supinated at the joint. This would be related to the posterior tibial muscle, the triceps muscle group, possibly the deltoid ligaments, and the anterior tibial muscle. They can also be caused by a relative contractural state of the peroneus longus muscle as this would plantarflex the first ray markedly which would cause the foot to be maximally supinated in the rearfoot when a child is ambulatory. This is one point which has been grossly overlooked in the past literature where they consider the peroneals as being a common unit; they are not. And the peroneus longus can definitely be a supinator of the talocalcaneal joint when weight-bearing.

(Figure 6). Here is a radiograph demonstrating a marked varus twist in the os calcis producing a varus rearfood deformity.

(Figure 7). A varus rearfoot including the whole foot radiographically in a 4-month-old child.

(Figure 8). A varus rearfoot bilaterally in an 8-year-old child.

The next level we shall talk about is the classical level that has been most understood throughout the years, and that is the equinus of the ankle. An equinus deformity ankle is a deformity between the talus and the tibialfibular unit. It can be positional related to a contractural state or an abnormal shortness of the triceps muscle group, or the whole posterior muscle group, and or the posterior capsule. It can be structural, related to flattening deformity of the talus trochlea which allows no more ankle dorsiflexion.

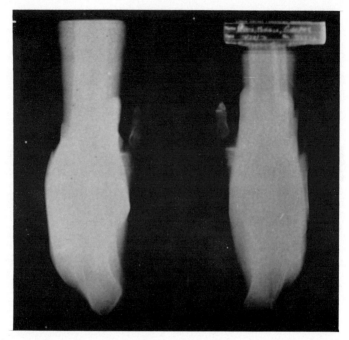

Figure 6.

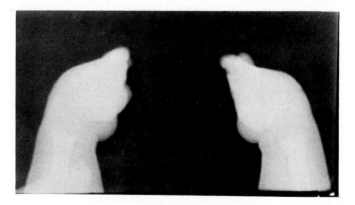

Figure 7.

(Figure 9). A radiograph of an equinus which is positional but fixed related to the posterior structures at that joint, from a lateral view.

(Figure 10). The same ankle as was demonstrated previously under maximum dorsiflexion stress showing range of excursion allowed by posterior structures at the tibial-talar joint.

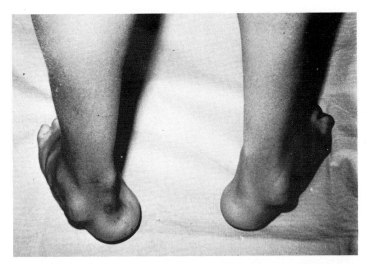

Figure 8.

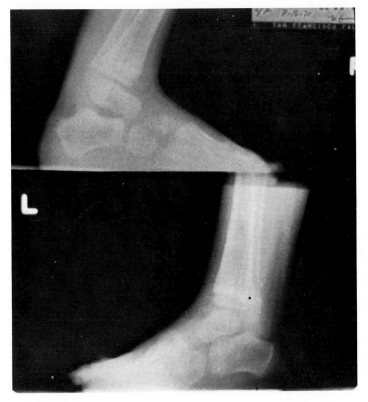

Figure 9.

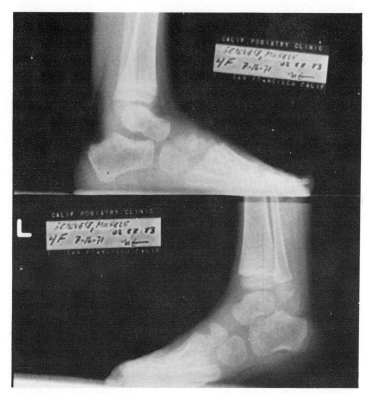

Figure 10.

(Figure 11). An equinus in a 6-month-old child.

Our next series demonstrates the typical equinovarus deformity in its full ramification. Clinically, its appearance at age 3 days with the deformity being present at all levels with a combination positional-structural deformity at each level.

(Figure 12). Clinically once again is a view at 3 days.

(Figure 13). A closeup of the foot at that stage.

(Figure 14). An x-ray of the foot at that stage.

(Figure 15). A foot following six months of casting on the foot, demonstrating the migration that has occurred at the Lisfranc joint, at the calcaneal cuboid, talonavicular joint with which the talonavicular joint is not completely corrected and the talocalcaneal joint which is not completely corrected.

(Figure 16). Clinically, here is a foot which had received multiple casting corrections prior to age four where the element of equino varus rearfoot adductus at the midtarsal and Lisfranc joints was still present.

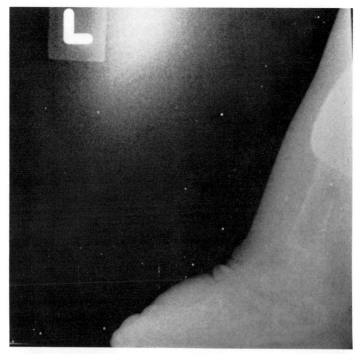

Figure 11.

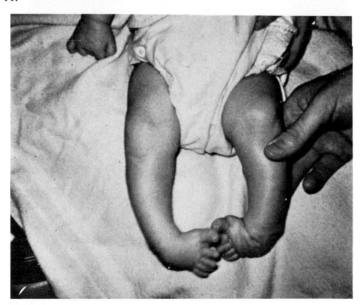

Figure 12.

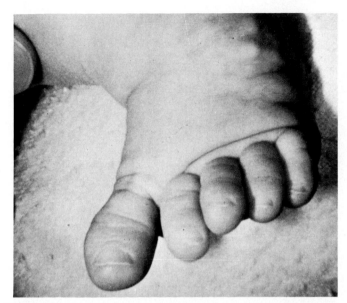

Figure 13.

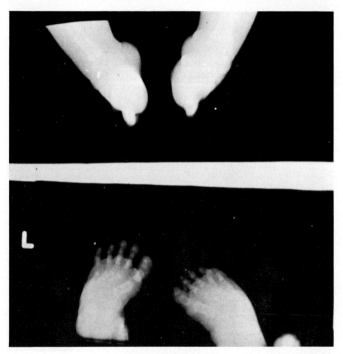

Figure 14.

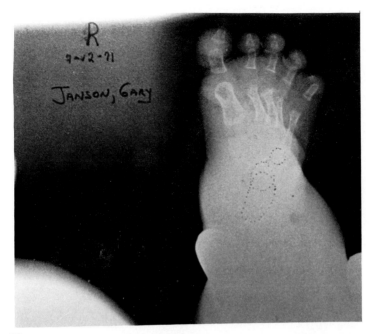

Figure 15.

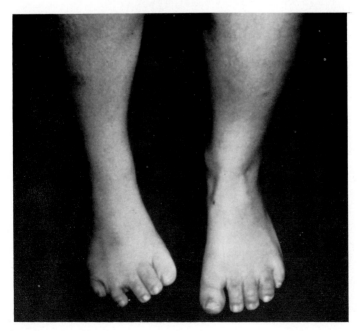

Figure 16.

(Figure 17). A view of a foot of a boy 8-years-old who demonstrates a typical equinovarus clubfoot position; however, this is neuromuscular in origin as the boy has progressive peroneal atrophy.

(Figure 18). The same foot from behind.

(Figure 19). Our last demonstration is of a person who had received multiple care for an equinovarus rearfoot deformity until present age 10. The rearfoot structure on observation appeared fairly good. The foot could dorsiflex at the ankle joint beyond 90 degrees, which was adequate. The foot appeared to be slightly more pronated to the ground than the other, which was not an abnormal finding. However, when we looked at the medial side of the foot we could see that there was a marked bulge at the talonavicular joint.

(Figure 20). Clinically, this view demonstrated only mild pronatory luxation. Looking at the foot from back to front however, we could see a marked varus forefoot.

(Figure 21). This was apparently related to the fact that the posterior tibial muscle had been detached and moved through the tibialfibular membrane to the dorsum of the foot to make the posterior tibia and ankle dorsiflexor.

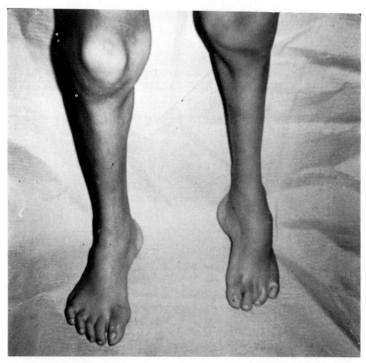

Figure 17.

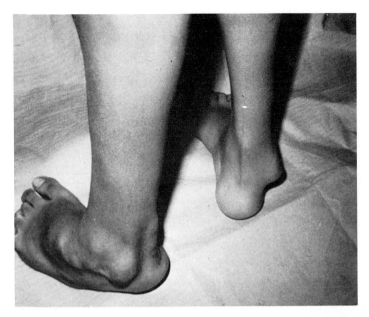

Figure 18.

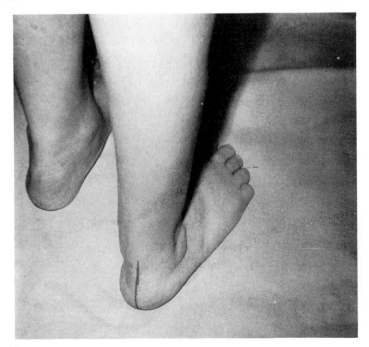

Figure 19.

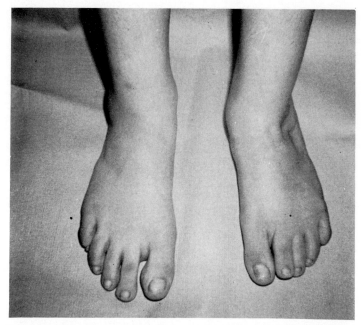

Figure 20.

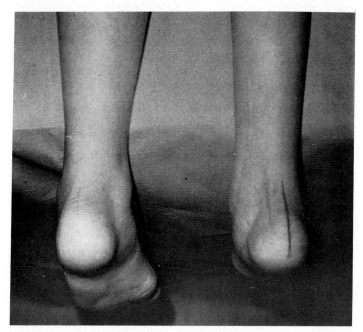

Figure 21.

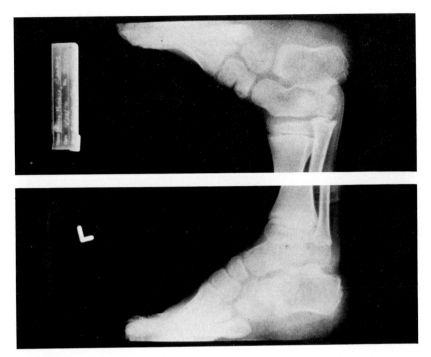

Figure 22.

(Figure 22). On this x-ray we see the complete dorsal location of the navicular to the talus which is progressive. The patient is gradually dislocating further and further and will require eventual arthrodesis.

The judgment of the musculature affecting any given joint has to be considered not only its effect on the joint but its antagonists, including the reaction of the ground.

This patient would have been better off only lengthening the posterior tibial muscle but leaving it.

VIII. Anesthesia

Local Infiltration Anesthesia

Robert E. Weinstock

In the past 13 years at Grand Community Hospital in Detroit, more than 50,000 different surgical procedures have been performed with use of lidocaine hydrochloride (Xylocaine) 1% or 2%, and 90-95% of these have been performed with Xylocaine with epinephrine. It has been noted by the American Heart Association that persons with cardiac (not vascular) insufficiencies should be given Xylocaine with epinephrine rather than Xylocaine plain because the primary pharmacologic action of Xylocaine is vasodilation. If a vasodilator is used in someone with cardiac insufficiency, peripheral vasoconstriction as a demand mechanism is created because of the vasodilation. So if Xylocaine with epinephrine is used two things occur: (1) absorption of the anesthetic into the general system is retarded and (2) the amount of peripheral epinephrine that is produced as a normal response of the body is greatly reduced. In other words, if you are going to give plain anesthesia, the response of the body itself to the plain anesthesia, in the amount of epinephrine produced, is much more than you could possibly give with Xylocaine with epinephrine. The safe limit of Xylocaine with epinephrine is 500 milligrams per surgical procedure. In other words, if you are using 2% Xylocaine, it is 25 cc, because it is 20 milligrams per cc; if you are using 1% Xylocaine with epinephrine, or plain, it is 50 cc.

Generally, Xylocaine with epinephrine is not harmful to normal healthy individuals. However, persons with vascular impairment should not have epinephrine. In our hospital 90% of the foot surgery is performed under local anesthesia using Xylocaine with epinephrine.

As to the type of needle we generally use, the average needle is 25 gauge, 1" long which is used in 95% of our local anesthesia cases; Xylocaine, or lidocaine hydrochloride, 1%, or 2% with epinephrine in most cases is the common local anesthetic.

Some persons tell you that they are allergic to a local anesthesia. I would suggest going a few steps further in your investigation. Many reasons could be given for passing out in a doctor or dentist's office after Xylocaine injection. In

---

Robert E. Weinstock, D.P.M., *Research Director, Grand Community Hospital Detroit, Michigan.*

testing for sensitivity to Xylocaine the fastest way is to drop Xylocaine in the corner of the patient's eye. You can see an immediate reaction with redness and streakiness if sensitivity to Xylocaine is present. An intradermal injection of 1-2 minims of Xylocaine (with epinephrine) will also elicit a sensitivity reaction.

I would like to review local anesthesia from the aspect of its administration. In doing so we will give you another anatomy lesson.

Figure 1. One of the most important things in local anesthesia is knowing which nerve to anesthetize when you are going to perform a surgical procedure. For example, adequate anesthesia for resection of the fifth metatarsal head involves the following: the sural nerve innervates the lateral side of the fifth metatarsal head. An anterior tibial block, or a superficial peroneal block, would

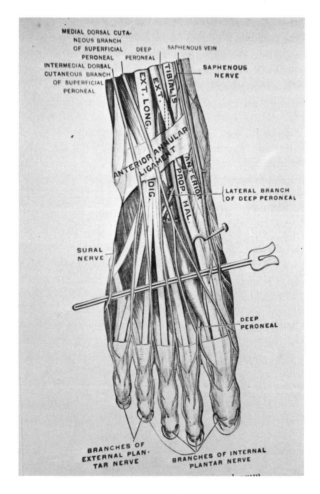

Figure 1.

not be sufficient for the dorsum of the fifth metatarsal. If you give anesthesia for a deep peroneal block you will get anesthesia of the adjacent sides of the first and second toe and part of the tibial aspect of the hallux. You can trace it yourself, from where it says "deep peroneal," which is also known as the anterior tibial; the nerve goes down between the first and second toes, and also the tibial side of the first toe. However, block of the superficial peroneal will anesthetize the adjacent sides of the fourth and fifth toes, fourth and third toes. The deep peroneal also sends up a branch to the second and third toes. According to Adriani, his injection for the deep peroneal, or anterior tibial nerve, is between the tibialis anterior tendon and the extensor hallucis longus tendon at the level of the ankle. We believe that it is better to inject at the ankle level above the malleoli so that both superficial and deep peroneal nerves may be anesthetized. The saphenous nerve is not very important unless one is doing work at the base of the first metatarsal where a local field block is usually employed.

Figure 2. The branching of the common peroneal nerve is illustrated, showing how it wraps around the head of the fibula and supplies the deep and superficial peroneal nerves. A common peroneal nerve block is used in lateral ankle sprains, or where you want to tape the foot in a particular position as in peroneal spastic flat floot, or in injuries to the peroneal nerve where complete relaxation of those particular areas is desirable.

Figure 3. The tibial nerve and the common peroneal nerve arise in the posterior aspect of the leg and behind the knee. The common peroneal nerve wraps around the head of the fibula and comes anterior, the fibular nerve comes down along the posterior aspect of the leg and then wraps around the media malleolus; at this point, it is the posterior tibial nerve.

Figure 4. This shows the distribution of the tibial and posterior tibial nerve into the medial and lateral plantar nerves. The fourth toe is the only toe that is innervated by both the medial and lateral plantar nerves. DuVries indicates that the significance of an intermetatarsal neuroma in the third metatarsal interspace is because of a conjoined nerve at that point, which would be a branch of the medial and lateral plantar nerves. I think that is why we see a neuroma more often in that particular area than in any other. You can see by the distribution of the nerves how the sole is innervated by the medial and lateral plantar nerves, the saphenous nerve, the tibial and sural nerves. It is sufficient to obtain anesthesia in the plantar surface of the foot to anesthetize the tibial, and posterior tibial, nerves.

Figure 5. This is a practical demonstration for the injection of a hallux. For this we use a 3 cc syringe to automatically limit the amount of local anesthetic to be used. More problems are caused by vasoconstriction due to too much volume of injected fluid than by the use of Xylocaine with epinephrine. The important part of the anesthesia is the proper distribution of the chemical, not

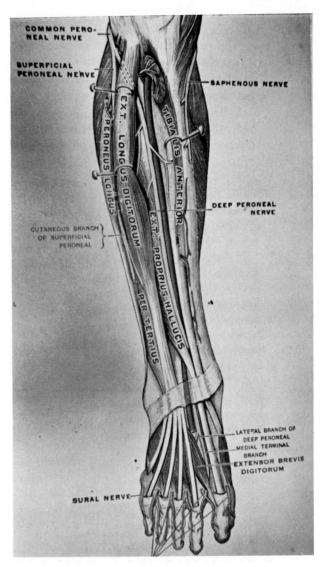

Figure 2.

the amount used. A wheal is raised with ¼ cc along the fibular aspect of the
hallux and then proceed in a plantarwise direction (Fig. 6) as you deposit
anesthetic toward the plantar aspect of the toe, putting about 1 cc in that area,
and then go across the dorsum of the the toe with about ¾ cc.

Figure 7. Please note the white area of the little wheal; this was done from
the dorsum of the toe. In this way the patient doesn't feel the second injection

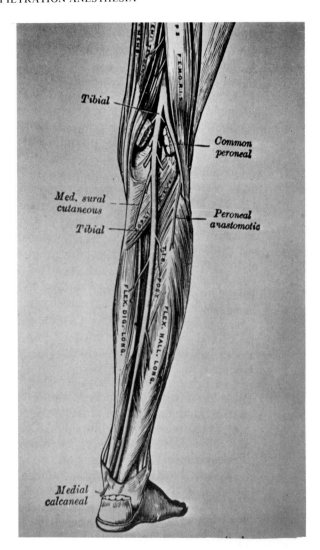

Figure 3.

of the needle; and then you go across the plantar aspect of the toe with about ¾ cc. You now have sufficient anesthesia, combining these two injections, to perform almost any type of surgery that is contemplated on the hallux.

Figure 8. Posterior tibial injections can be given in several areas. This one is given directly above the level of the medial malleolus. The posterior tibial nerve is just posterior to the posterior tibial artery, the injection is made about ¼ " posterior to the palpable pulse of this artery.

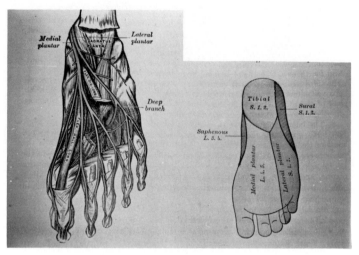

Figure 4.

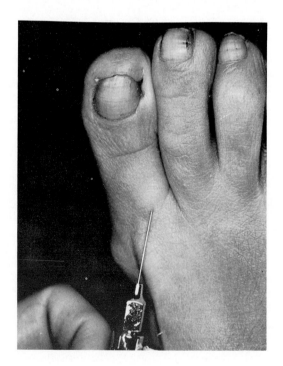

Figure 5.

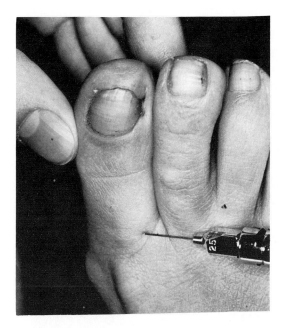

Figure 6.

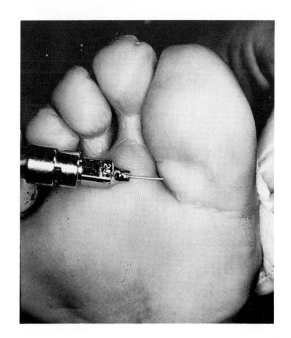

Figure 7.

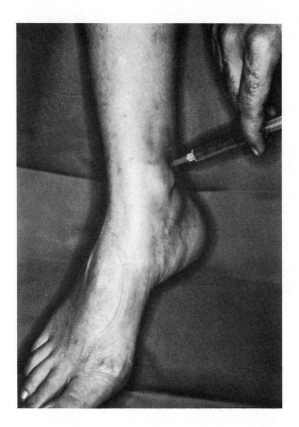

Figure 8.

Figure 9. In this injection, of the deep and superficial peroneal nerves I usually use about 5 cc, fanning out in either direction. Adriani's description of an injection of an interior tibial nerve is as I described; between the anterior tibial tendon and the extensor hallucis longus; this of course will only give you anesthesia of the first and second toes and a part of the third toe.

Figure 10. We give our injection at the level of the ankle, fibular to the palpable anterior tibial pulse; we inject down between the malleoli with about 1 cc of anesthetic and then fan out in either direction; fanning out in the fibular direction you pick up the superficial peroneal nerve, in the tibial direction – the deep peroneal nerve. This injection will give you dorsal anesthesia of the first, second, third, fourth, and one-half of the fifth toe, but not its lateral side.

Figure 11. The sural nerve can be approached from the posterior direction; it is uncommonly used and included only for didactic review.

Figure 12. In performing a common peroneal block, you palpate for the head of the fibula and inject about 3 cc of anesthetic subcutaneously. This is the

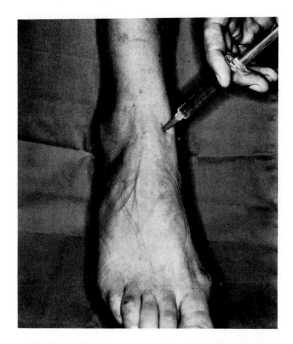

Figure 9.

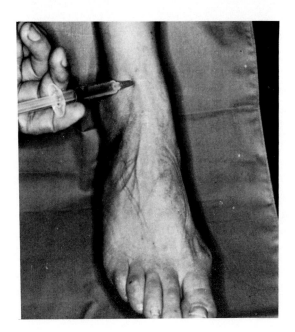

Figure 10.

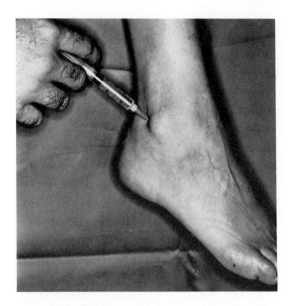

Figure 11.

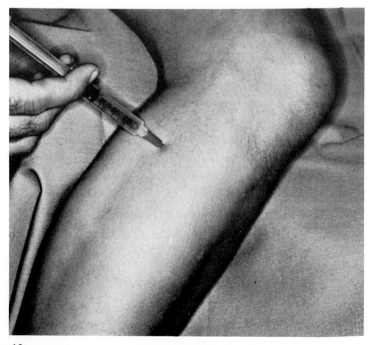

Figure 12.

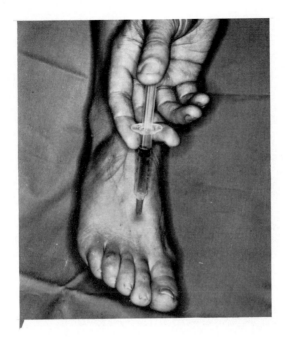

Figure 13.

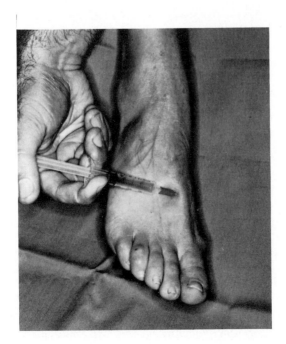

Figure 14.

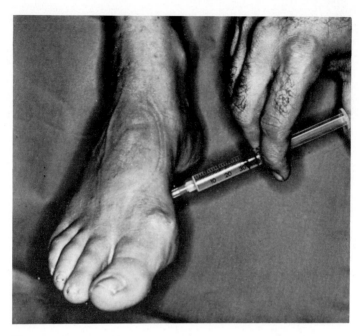

Figure 15.

area which nerve is commonly responsible for the "falling asleep" of your leg after sitting for some time with your legs crossed; due to the crushing of common peroneal nerve by the head of the fibula.

Figure 13. The most popular injection for bunion surgery by those who don't want to do block anesthesia is called the Mayo block. Actually, this is a ring of anesthetic at the base of the first metatarsal. In this injection we prefer to use a 25 gauge, 1½" needle (Becton-Dickinson disposable); about 2 cc of anesthestic is deposited along the shaft of the first metatarsal, (Figure 14) and then you inject in a tibial direction with about 2 cc in the dorsum of the foot.

Figure 15. Another 2 cc is injected across the plantar aspect. In all, the Mayo block takes about 5-6 cc. When I use this type of anesthesia I inject anesthetic also into the area of the fibular sesamoid and along the line of incision on the dorsum of the first metatarsal phalangeal joint.

I did not review digital anesthesia because this is just a matter of injecting from the dorsum in a V-shape to either side of a toe, using 1½-2½ cc depending on the size of the digit.

The important part of the anesthetic technique is not to give too much anesthesia in a confined area but to give sufficient anesthesia in the correct area. For example, 3 cc of anesthetic in a hallux may not anesthetize the toe, if the anesthetic is not properly distributed.

Summary

The use of lidocaine hydrochloride with epinephrine, 1:100,000 is not contraindicated in foot surgery, if used in patients with normal vascularization, in the correct dosage.

Nitrous Oxide Analgesia in Podiatry

Mark H. Feldman

Introduction

Nitrous oxide analgesia (NOA) (relative analgesia) is a chemically induced, altered psychological state which eliminates the fear, anxiety, apprehension and, partially, the pain of the podiatric experience. It results from the psychological and physiological effects of low alveolar concentrations of nitrous oxide in combination with oxygen.[2]

Purpose of Analgesia

Nitrous oxide analgesia (relative analgesia) has as its primary purpose the elimination of fear and anxiety. What do these terms really mean? Fear is attached to an external object or situation. This means that people fear an animal, fear an airplane, fear the hospital, or fear the podiatrist. Anxiety, on the other hand, seems to be generated from an internal threat and usually the patient becomes nervous without really knowing what he is nervous about. It is generated from something or someone that you really cannot do anything about. Our fears and anxieties are different and their manifestations are different.

Of secondary importance in the use of relative analgesia is the relief of pain. It is true that the pain threshold is increased and this certainly helps but even if this were not the case, Nitrous oxide would still be very useful to the podiatrist.

The gag reflex is obtunded. Long appointments do not bother the patient as much since he is relaxed. The memory of discomfort is reduced. It eliminates the anticipation of discomfort.

Benefits to the patient:

1. Eliminates fear and anxiety.

2. Pain is obtunded when the local anesthetic is administered. The dread of the injection is eliminated.

3. Eliminates the anticipation of pain and discomfort.

Mark H. Feldman, B.S., D.P.M., *Doctors Hospital, Tucker, Ga.*

4. More relaxed for longer appointments.

5. The memory of the discomfort is reduced or obliterated.

The purpose of this paper is to evaluate the use and effectiveness of NOA when used in combination with local anesthesia to make the podiatric surgical experience more pleasant for the patient. This then would obviate the need for oral, i.m. or i.v. sedatives or barbiturates as pre-operative medications.

This analgesic method would allow for complete control of the patient's consciousness by the doctor and allow complete recovery immediately post-operatively.

The paper will introduce the podiatrist to the concept of NOA and to illustrate its possible place in the practice of podiatric medicine and surgery. The paper is based on the personal experiences of the author made possible by the administration of NOA to 25 patients, 10 of whom were practicing podiatrists.

Definitions

1. *Analgesia:* loss of sensibility to pain. It is literally without pain; the loss of pain usually due to drug administration, but *without loss of consciousness.*
2. *Anesthesia:* loss of sensation in a part or in the body generally; with the loss of consciousness.
3. *Relative Analgesia:* an induced altered psychological state which reduces fear and pain of expected procedures.
4. *Amnesia:* loss of memory.
5. *Euphoria:* a state of mind; a feeling that all is well.
6. *Ataraxia:* complete calmness and peace of mind.

Physiology of Respiration[1]

Before we begin to understand the physiology of nitrous oxide, we must have a working background of normal respiration. Respiration is the gaseous exchange of oxygen from the air to the cells of the body, and the carrying of carbon dioxide from the body cells back into the atmospheric air. This definition can be broken down into external respiration, which is the gaseous exchange between the air and the blood by way of the lungs, and internal respiration, which is the exchange of gases between the blood and the body cells.

The external respiration consists of a conducting portion which is the anatomical dead space – the nasopharynx, oropharynx, pharynx, larynx, trachea, and the bronchi – and the ventilating portion which is the lungs. Internal respiration is made up of the transportation portion and intracellular respiration. The transportation system is the plasma and red cells of the blood. Intracellular respiration is the exchange of oxygen and carbon dioxide between the blood and the body cells.

The mechanics of respiration involves differences in the pressure within the lungs and the atmospheric pressure. In breathing there is an inspiratory effort and an expiratory phase. There are four phases to the inspiratory effort:

1. A nervous impulse causes the diaphragm and the intercostal muscles to contract.
2. Because of the muscle contraction there is an enlargement in the thoracic cage.
3. The cage enlargement causes an increase in the interpleural negative pressure forcing the lungs to increase in size and thus capacity. This produces a transitional increase in the intrapulmonic negative pressure.
4. Through the anatomical dead space or conducting portion the air from the atmosphere enters the lungs until the intrapulmonic and the atmospheric pressures are equal.

The expiratory phase of the expelling of the air also has four steps:

1. When the lungs have expanded to their normal limits there is stimulation of many stretch receptors in the visceral pleura which causes the diaphragm and the intercostals to reflex (Herring-Breurer reflex).
2. The relaxation of the muscles causes a decrease in the dimensions of the thoracic cage.
3. A decrease in dimension causes an increase in pressure upon the intrapleural surfaces, and this raises the pressure within the lungs.
4. The conducting portion again conducts the gases into the air until the intrapulmonic and atmospheric pressures are equal.

Control of Respiration

Control of respiration can be chemical, neurological, or by voluntary means. Neural controls are centered in the medulla where the inspiratory and expiratory centers are located. The pneumotoxic center, which gives breathing a rhythmic pattern, is located in the pons. Inspiration is started by the stimulation of the muscles in inspiration by impulses from the inspiratory center. When the lungs become extended, the stretch receptors are stimulated, sending afferent nerve impulses by way of the vagus to the brain where the impulses inhibit further inspiration (Herring-Breurer reflex).

Chemoreceptors are cells located in the aortic and common carotid arteries which can help neural regulation of respiration when there is lack of oxygen in the system. These bodies are stimulated when the arterial oxygen concentration falls below 92% saturation. Stimulation to these bodies increases the depth of respiration rather than the rate.

Pressoreceptors are sinus formations which are located at the junction of the internal and external carotid arteries, and at the arch of the aorta. When these vessels are stretched because of an increase in blood pressure, there are impulses sent to the expiratory center to inhibit expiration and to decrease the depth and rate of respiration.

Peripheral pain can cause an increase in respiration through the peripheral afferent nerve fibers. Visceral pain can cause a decrease in respiration.

The chemical control has an overall influence over the neural and voluntary control of respiration. The respiratory center is extremely sensitive to the carbon dioxide tension in the blood. A minimum increase above normal stimulates the respiratory center, which will increase the depth of respiration. A decrease in carbon dioxide tension can cause apnea. Pulmonary ventilation and carbon dioxide levels in the arterial blood are the prime factors in maintaining the acid-base balance of the body. When the carbon dioxide level is increased, the increase in ventilation reduces the carbon dioxide content of the arterial blood, and a reduced carbon dioxide level will decrease ventilation, permitting the carbon dioxide tension to increase.

Oxygen tension in the arterial blood has little effect upon the respiratory center. An increase in tension has practically no effect on ventilation, whereas a sufficient lack in oxygen concentration will depress the respiratory center and nervous tissue. This is a significant factor to remember when administering analgesia. In severe respiratory depression, either caused by lack of oxygen or an anesthetic agent, neither drugs nor carbon dioxide will be enough to stimulate the respiratory center. These patients must be ventilated so that the center will eventually respond to the carbon dioxide levels and reflex stimuli.

The hydrogen ion concentration in the blood has an effect on respiration, but not as drastic an effect as carbon dioxide. A low pH will increase the rate and depth of respiration. Acidosis can increase the ventilatory rate.

Voluntary control is only possible within certain limits. It is possible to hyperventilate, and to increase the duration of apnea. Respiration is altered voluntarily when a person sings, coughs, and whistles. This type of control is managed by impulses from the motor cortex to the respiratory center. Voluntary control can only be affected insofar as the chemical control permits.

The ventilating portion of the respiratory system is concerned with the exchanges of gases between the alveoli of the lungs and the bloodstream. This exchange depends on the differences of the partial pressures of the gases involved and on the physical condition of the alveoli. The rate and speed of which the gases diffuse can be altered: they may be decreased by pulmonary edema or other diseases of the lung.

The external portion of the respiratory system gets the air into the blood and the internal system gets the oxygen into the tissues and cells and returns the carbon dioxide.

Oxygen is carried by the blood – 10 ml/100 ml – it is in chemical combination with hemoglobin, and 0.3 ml/100 ml – is in plasma. Because of the differences in pressure gradients, the oxygen diffuses into the alveoli, into the blood, and into the tissue and cells. Arterial blood contains 19 ml of $O_2/100$ ml and venous blood contains 14 ml of $O_2/100$ ml; the difference being absorbed by the tissues.

Carbon dioxide is carried in the venous blood as sodium bicarbonate in the plasma, carbaminohemoglobin, carbonic acid in plasma, and potassium bicarbonate in the red blood cells. This complicated action of carbon dioxide is known as the chloride shift. Because of the differences in the partial pressures, 5-15 ml of $CO_2/100$ ml of blood is taken away from the tissue and into the blood.

The final stage of respiration is the exchange of oxygen and carbon dioxide between the capillaries, tissues, and cells. This is the prime function of respiration. The oxygen concentration in the blood is greater than the concentration of oxygen in the tissue and cells, thus diffusion takes place. The tissue and cells will use oxygen at a rate partially dependent upon the activity of the tissue. The greater the uptake of oxygen the greater the give-off of carbon dioxide. As oxygen, carbon dioxide will diffuse from an area of greater concentration to an area of lesser concentration. The chloride shift occurs because the membrane of the red cells is permeable only to bicarbonate and chloride anion. The chloride shift enables the blood to increase the carbon dioxide carrying powers of the blood plasma. As the blood gives up oxygen, its efficiency as a carrier of carbon dioxide is increased. The arterial blood, having given up oxygen and taken up carbon dioxide from the tissues, is transformed into venous blood. The blood is returned to the right atrium and ventricles to the pulmonary arteries and to the lungs. It is in the lungs that it is reconverted into arterial blood by the ventilating portion of the external respiratory system.

Physiology of Respiration with Reference to
Anesthesia and Analgesia[6]

Anesthetic agents (of which nitrous oxide is one — it is a 15% effective anesthetic agent) can alter both the sensitivity and threshold of the respiratory center to the carbon dioxide in the blood. Carbon dioxide can build up to depressing levels before an oxygen deficiency is noticeable. Oxygen has very limited stimulating power on the center, but a lack of oxygen (hypoxia) can depress the center so that it will not respond to the normal stimulating mechanisms. So when an anesthetic or analgesic is given, sufficient oxygen must be administered so that the respiratory center can respond to the normal stimuli.

Nitrous oxide must have sufficient concentration in the bloodstream before it can affect the central nervous system. The first type of tissue to be affected is the brain, and the effect must be controlled in a sufficient manner so that the other body tissues aren't affected to any great extent. The brain tissue is more susceptible to nitrous oxide because it receives a higher percentage of the circulating blood volume. It is possible to depress certain parts of the brain so that some of the vital signs are depressed in different stages, thus the different stages of anesthesia.

Nitrous oxide is carried to all of the tissues of the body in proportion to that tissue's volume blood supply. Since the tissue and the cells have a high content of water, the effectiveness of an anesthetic on the tissue is partially dependent upon its solubility in water.

Among the prevalent theories on the action of anesthetic agents is the lipoidal, or Overton-Meyer Theory. A drug or a gas has a specific affinity for fats, and this affinity is related to the agent's absorption. The brain has a high content of lipoid tissue, which may be why nitrous oxide affects the central nervous system before there is any other significant effect on other body tissues.

Body position is important in the use of nitrous oxide because if the patient is reclined, most of the lung capacities and volumes are decreased. Any factor which decreases the vital capacity of the lungs could reduce the ability of the lungs to expand. This is an important fact to remember when administering nitrous oxide to patients with TB, emphysema, asthma, carcinomas, bronchitis, or pleurisy. Vital capacity is reduced in any heart disease. This can cause vascular congestion in the lungs, because the excessive fluid in the lungs will decrease pulmonary compliance.

If oxygen has been supplied to the body tissues in no less a percentage than in normal atmospheric air (20.9%), the cells of the central nervous system are restored to normal function after the use of nitrous oxide. Circulation time of the blood from the lungs to the brain to the lungs is thirty seconds. This is why a nitrous oxide-oxygen analgesia patient can experience effects in a short period of time. Nitrous oxide is not absorbed by the red blood cells. The atmospheric air that we breathe is about 79% nitrogen, and approximately the same amount is in the lungs. It is the nitrogen that is replaced in the lungs, not the oxygen. The blood is only able to take up about 1.7 volume per cent of nitrogen, but it can take up to 26 volume per cent of nitrous oxide. This fifteen times greater solubility of nitrous oxide over nitrogen also helps explain the difference of effect on the tissue and the central nervous system.

The Pharmacology of Nitrous Oxide[2]

An anesthetic can cause depression of the respiration. The ideal anesthetic would depress respiration the least and the cortex the most. Nitrous oxide-oxygen analgesia has often been compared to 10-15 mg of morphine. Nitrous oxide's action with the bloodstream is a pure physical one. There is no chemical combination with any of the tissues. It is non-irritating to the mucous membranes of the anatomical dead space. Nitrous oxide does not replace oxygen in the alveoli, but replaces nitrogen. There is no detrimental effect on the heart, liver or the kidney when it is used with oxygen. Nitrous oxide is excreted from the lungs unchanged.

No known chemical reaction involving nitrous oxide occurs on its inhalation. Its pharmacologic actions occur mainly in the central nervous system and are mild.

Elimination. The elimination of nitrous oxide takes place largely through the lungs. A small amount of excretion occurs also through skin, sweat glands, urine, and intestinal gas.

Cerebrospinal Fluid. There is no change in the composition or volume of the cerebrospinal fluid attrributed to nitrous oxide.

Cough Reflex. When used as general anesthesia, nitrous oxide causes the cough reflex to be suppressed only to a moderate extent. When used as relative analgesia, there is no suppression of the cough reflex.

The Circulatory System. Nitrous oxide does not cause any change in heart rate or cardiac output, nor any changes in arterial pressure or venous pressure. Cutaneous venodilation does occur, and this effect has been used to facilitate venipuncture when veins are not visible before induction. The blood volume and composition are not changed except after more than 24 to 48 hours of continuous administration in concentrations greater than 25 per cent nitrous oxide. Under these conditions the white blood count is decreased. It returns to normal upon cessation of administration of nitrous oxide.

The Respiratory System. The sensitivity of the nasolaryngotracheal area is markedly reduced, and the sense of smell is decreased. The latter effect has made nitrous oxide popular as an induction agent with the use of more irritating anesthetic agents. Nitrous oxide is much less toxic than other inhalation anesthesia drugs.

The Gastrointestinal System. Esophageal, gastric, and intestinal peristalses are not affected, and gastrointestinal secretions continue. Gas in bowel may be replaced by nitrous oxide as a result of the denitrogenation process. The hepatic and pancreatic functions are unaffected.

The Genitourinary System. There is no change in kidney function, ureteral peristalses, bladder tone, or urine formation, nor any effect on the genital organs.

Metabolism. Nitrous oxide does not appear either to stimulate nor to depress metabolism, as is evidenced by oxygen uptake.

Stages of Analgesia[2]

Plane 1 – *Parasthesia*

The sympathetic nervous system goes into action and the patient feels a "tingling" sensation usually in the fingers, lips, toes, or tongue. No decrease in pain or fear occurs at this stage.

Plane 2 – *Vasomotor*

The sympathetic nervous system is still active and causes a "warm feeling" usually all over the body. Usually the head and legs are affected first. The legs and head or hands may feel "heavy." The patient using N_2O for the first time may get a little nervous here. He may state that he cannot breathe, or his chest feels heavy or his heart is beating fast. All that is necessary is reassurance. The patient can still see, hear and talk.

Plane 3 – *Drift*

The subcortical areas of the brain now come into play. The patient may feel as if he were light as a feather or is floating off the chair. The feeling of europhoria begins. The patient is now more relaxed and calm. The pain threshold is increased or, in other words, his pain is decreased. The peripheral vision may become blurred and the blink reflex is diminished. As you talk to your patient your voice may seem distant to him. At this stage it is important to keep talking to the patient.

Plane 4 – *Dream*

The limbic and reticular activating systems come into play. The patient generally closes his eyes and shows only limited awareness. The patient can still hear but usually he does not talk as much as before. His speech is slow and deliberate. Many have dreams of various types. There is complete relaxation. Vital signs are stable.

Plane 5 – *Pre-Excitement – Total Analgesia*

There is total amnesia. The patient may laugh suddenly or try to get up from the chair, or try to take the nosepiece off. He may grunt or moan. The facial muscles, especially the muscles of mastication, become rigid. There may be generalized muscle contractions. The pulse generally is increased as may be the blood pressure. The patient is totally unresponsive to all questions. Note the two biggest things associated with this plane are that the patient is unresponsive to your questions and that his mouth will not stay open on its own. These are important points.

TABLE 1. The Stages of Anesthesia and Analgesia

Stage I					Stage II	Stage III	Stage IV
Plane 1	Plane 2	Plane 3	Plane 4	Plane 5			
Parasthesia	Vasomotor	Drift	Dream	Pre-Excitement	Delirium	Surgical Anesthesia 4 planes	Respiratory Paralysis
	Relative Analgesia			Total Analgesia			
						From Langa[2] and Carnow[5]	

Differences Between Analgesia and Anesthesia[2]

Relative Analgesia	*General Anesthesia*
1. Patient is awake, can hear, talk and can comply with directions: hence, easy to judge depth.	Patient is unconscious. Depth can be judged by clinical signs only.
2. No risk involved, no case of a death with analgesia only.	More risk involved.
3. Nausea and vomiting rare.	Nausea and vomiting fairly frequent.
4. Patient is awake and the cough reflex is present. The gag reflex is obtunded making dental treatment easier.	Patient is asleep and the cough reflex gone. Aspiration more of a hazard.
5. A higher % of O_2 used.	A lower % of O_2 used.
6. Used routinely in dentistry.	Rarely used in dentistry.
7. Recovery rapid.	Recovery slow.
8. Mouth props not necessary.	Mouth props needed.
9. No premedication necessary.	Premedication used.
10. Easily used in podiatric office.	Primarily used in hospital.
11. Patient acceptance good.	Patient acceptance poor.
12. Need not always have empty stomach.	Need empty stomach.
13. Patient can alter depth voluntarily hence feels as if he has control of situation.	Patient is unconscious and cannot alter depth. He has no control of situation.

Analgesia: The Stage of Relative Analgesia[5]

In the stage of relative analgesia the patient's threshold to pain, cold, warmth, and light touch is raised. Although the special senses may be partly obtunded and a sensation of numbness is described, superficial and deep reflexes remain active and the sensorium remains clear. Consciousness is impaired only to a slight degree. These changes may be demonstrated by placing the patient in the analgesic state and then stimulating the skin with a sharp instrument. There is a quick withdrawal from the stimulus. However, depending on the degree of analgesia relative to the intensity of the stimulus, the patient may not interpret the stimulus as painful. Although it may evoke a reflex and the subject is aware of being stimulated, the reaction to and the intepretation of the severity of the pain are dulled. Pain relief of this sort without abolition of reflexes is inadequate for major surgery, but it is highly suitable for podiatric injections, especially when the fear-eliminating properties of this stage are kept in mind.

The Signs and Symptoms of Relative Analgesia

What does a patient look like and what does he feel when in the stage of relative analgesia? A patient in this stage is conscious, and his facial expression is that of a conscious individual. His respiration is normal and smooth, and his muscles are relaxed. The pupils are normal and they contract normally to light. The conjunctiva is sensitive, there is no rolling of the eyeballs, the eyelids do not resist opening and they wink when touched. The patient's pulse rate is normal, as are his blood pressure and the color of his skin.

After breathing nitrous oxide and oxygen for 30 to 40 seconds, the patient may become aware of first the taste of the gases and then the odor. The odor of nitrous oxide may best be described as a mild ethereal odor. Its mildness and lack of irritating qualities make it pleasant and easy to take for most people, a fact of tremendous importance to the dentist, because it means more ready acceptance of analgesia by the patient, especially when first introduced.

The first subjective symptom may be a tingling sensation in the toes, the fingertips, or the tip of the tongue. Often a patient will describe a tingly or numb sensation in the lips. These symptoms are due to vasomotor excitation. Although these symptoms are fairly characteristic of the light analgesic state, all are not necessarily present at each administration. Then, too, the patient may not always be able to clearly distinguish them, especially when he has gone deeper into the analgesic stage. Operators new to the use of analgesia often use the absence of these symptoms as an indication that the analgesia is too light. The reverse may be true, however, for the patient may already be in the deep analgesic state. The best procedure when in doubt is to begin work on the patient. Since we are treating a conscious patient, his reaction, verbal or physical, will indicate his status.

The patient may experience diaphoresis as a result of a psychic disturbance during the state of altered consciousness. If desired, this can be prevented by premedication with belladonna.

As the patient gets deeper into the analgesic stage, he may feel a warm wave suffuse his entire body. He has a feeling of lethargy. Very often he experiences a humming, droning, or vibratory sensation throughout his body somewhat like the soft purring of a motor. At this time, the patient may also describe a feeling of heaviness or drowsiness, similar to light intoxication. His voice becomes throaty, losing its natural resonance. Normally the voice is projected through the head and nose; under analgesia the voice seems to acquire a peculiar, characteristic throaty tone.

Although the patient under analgesia is not unconscious, he is not fully awake. He knows something is going on about him, yet he is less aware of his surroundings and less concerned with what is taking place than normally. In spite of himself, he begins to experience a feeling of relaxation. He has a feeling of well-being, of safety, of euphoria. There is a feeling of being in a friendly atmosphere and of having a friend at hand should there be the need of one. He feels warm and comfortable, as if he were in a pleasant dream. Words reach him as form a great distance. He may hear the doctor ask a question, yet he may not readily respond because he thinks, "I know the doctor is asking me a question, but I can't be bothered answering. I feel too good to bother answering."

As the deeper phase of the relative analgesic stage is attained, pain disappears but recognition of touch and pressure is still present. Sounds come to the patient distinctly but more distantly. Sudden loud noises may bring him out of his pleasant euphoric state. If he attempts to lift his arm or leg, it will feel heavy and cumbersome, and he cannot fully control its movements. His thoughts very often wander far afield. He may engage in philosophical thoughts or mull over religious problems. He may attempt to solve some of the world's problems and be anxious to impart this knowledge to the doctor upon awakening. Usually, however, he is unable to do so; his memory of the immediate past is dim.

**TABLE 2. Signs of Relative Analgesia versus
Light Anesthesia**

	Relative Analgesia	*Light Anesthesia*
Respiration	Normal, Smooth	Superficial slow breathing, often irregular
	Inspiration of normal duration	Prolonged inspiration
	No phonation	Phonation due to reflexes of pain
	No holding of breath or grunting	Holding of breath, grunting
General Muscles	No movements, muscles relaxes	Purposeful movement or rigid muscles
	Facial expression of conscious individual	Facial expression of pain or semiconsciousness
	Nausea extremely rare	Nausea more frequent
	Pusposeful but delayed resistance as result of trauma	Reflex or purposeful resistance as result of trauma
Eye	Pupils normal, contract normally to light	Pupils large, contract to light actively
	Conjunctiva sensitive	Conjunctiva sensitive
	No rolling of eyeballs	Eyeballs roll quite rapidly
	Eyelids do not resist opening, wink when touched	Eyelids resist opening, wink when touched
Pulse Rate	Normal	Accelerated
Blood Pressure	Normal	Normal
Color of Skin	Normal	Pink or no change normally In anemics, no color change In plethorics, slight cyanosis

The Introduction of Analgesia to the Patient

This should include:

a. A description of the usual experiences a patient has under analgesia; namely, the parasthesia, vasomotor, drift and dream plateaus.

b. A description and view of the apparatus to be placed on the face of the patient; that is, the nosepiece or cannula.

c. An emphasis on the facts that the patient does not go to sleep and is completely ambulatory after he leaves the chair.

A patient analgesia information form that may be used follows:

A Note to My Patients About Podiatric Analgesia

The fear of surgical pain is so common that most patients avoid surgical treatment.

WHY?

Novocaine has been used since 1905 and does an excellent job of reducing and eliminating pain.

But how about anxiety, fear and tension? It doesn't eliminate these problems! And yet . . . it is the fear, as well as pain, that keeps 50% of the American population away from the Podiatrist.

So what can we do today? Today we use analgesia.

It was first used 125 years ago and is still being used for relaxation and comfort.

- What is analgesia?
- Can it be used for children and adults?
- When do you use it?

Analgesia is a pleasant refreshing gas which is inhaled through the nose and is used by both children and adults.

- You do not go to sleep.
- You are awake.
- You can talk and see.
- There are no after effects.

It helps you to relax, eliminates a good deal of the nervousness and fear, and therefore, helps you before, during, and after your podiatry visit. When novocaine is needed, you do not mind it at all . . . Of course, you may drive . . . and go about your usual activities after you leave the office.

Another form of patient education is a typical information sheet given to each patient.

"A lifetime of health, comfort, and function of the feet is within the reach of us all. This is realized through good home care and regular professional care. The greatest deterrent to regular podiatric care is the fear of pain. In view of this, it is our endeavor to remove pain and fear of pain during podiatric treatment. To this end we offer our patients a variety of pain relievers and sedatives, according to each individual's needs and desires. Novocaine was designed for one purpose, and it does this well. It eliminates pain. But it does not eliminate the tension and anxiety generally associated with podiatric surgery in the minds of many people.

In our opinion, the use of a sedative combination of nitrous oxide and oxygen is a most pleasant method of achieving our aim. We call this "analgesia." The pleasant gases are inhaled through the nose from a nasal inhaler. You start to feel warm and relaxed and completely free of tension and anxiety. At no time do you go to sleep — you are completely awake and cooperative at all times. Novocaine is needed in addition to the analgesia, but you won't mind it at all. There are no lingering after effects; following treatment, you may go about your usual business. We only ask you to wait 10-15 minutes in the waiting room before driving home. Analgesia is in no way compulsory, and you may request novocaine only, if you so desire.

There is no more important aspect of nitrous oxide analgesia than taking the time to discuss this totally new experience with your patients.

Techniques and Administration[2]

In this study the Fraser-Sweatman Quantiflex RA machine was used. This was after an investigation proved this machine to have the most "fail-safe" device and the readable accessibility of a positive pressure respirating apparatus as an optional feature.

Administration was begun by allowing the patient to breathe 100% oxygen at 3 L/min for two minutes to allow him to become accustomed to the fit of the nasal inhaler nosepiece. After two minutes 3 L/min of nitrous oxide and 3 L/min of oxygen were given for 3-5 minutes. Then 4 minutes of nitrous oxide with 3 L/min of oxygen were given for 3-5 minutes until Plane 4 of Stage I was reached by each patient.

At this point, one or more punctures into the plantar surface of the calcaneus with a #23 1½ inch needle were made.

It was felt that if each patient could tolerate this procedure without total awareness of the pain then the administration was successful.

Any time a patient experiences marked pain as evidenced by complete leg withdrawal or oral sounds the test was deemed a failure.

There were 25 patients, 15 males, 10 females, all adult. Twenty-two patients were deemed successful and three, failures. The failures were due to pre-op medication in one patient, and insufficient time allowed in the second and third.

There was one instance of vomiting and five instances of slight nausea with three instances of post-analgesia cephalgia.

The study is to be continued at the Outpatient Surgery Department of the Ohio College of Podiatric Medicine.

It is my opinion at this time that nitrous oxide analgesia is of considerable value in the relief of Surgical apprehension and, to a lesser degree, pain.

References

1. Guyton, Arthur C., M.D.: *Textbook of Medical Physiology*, Second Edition, W. B. Saunders Co., 1961.
2. Langa, Harry: *Relative Analgesia in Dental Practice*, W. B. Saunders Co., 1968.
3. Monheim, Leonard: *General Anesthesia in Dental Practice*, C. V. Mosby Co., 1964.
4. Silver, Sidney, and Fordham, Kenneth C.: *Analgesia*, 304 King of Prussia Road, Radnor, Pennsylvania, 19087.
5. Carnow, Ralph: Simplified Analgesia, in Kilpatrick's *Work Simplification in Dental Practice*, W. B. Saunders Co., 1969.
6. Eastwood, D. W. (Ed.): Clinical Anesthesia/Clinical Use of Nitrous Oxide, F. A. Davis Co., 1964.

Intravenous Regional Anesthesia

John J. McGlone

Intravenous regional anesthesia has been used for over 60 years. The procedure was first introduced by August Karl Gustuv Bier in 1908 and was employed on a limited scale in various parts of the world over the next 50 years. The main reason for its limited use was the necessity for a cutdown to deliver the anesthetic solution.[1] In 1931, Morrison in England gave a detailed account of his use of the method and it was he who first suggested the use of venipuncture, thus making the technique more practical.[2]

It was 1963 before Bier's technique received widespread attention. Holmes[3] published his results with the procedure and immediately it gained in popularity and use.

From March 1967 through April 1970, 62 patients whom we studied had podiatric surgery performed with the use of intravenous regional anesthesia. The distribution of the patients and the operative procedures are as follows:

1. **Sex.** Female, 49; male, 13.

2. **Age Span.** Twenty years through 75 years.

3. **Podiatric Procedures:** excision of Morton's neuroma, 23; McBride bunionectomy, 6; Keller bunionectomy, 5; Schede bunionectomy, 5; Du Vries plantar condylectomy, 4; medial sesamoidectomy, 4; tailor bunionectomy, 2; excision of ganglion, 2; excision of fibroma, 1; open reduction and internal fixation of fracture, 1; bone biopsy, 1; excision of bursa of tendo calcaneus, 1; excision of hemangioma, 1; surgical syndactylism, 1; correction of Dupuytren's contracture, 1; excision of rheumatoid nodule, 1; amputation of hallux, 1; Jones' suspension, 1; excision of foreign granuloma, 1.

Method

The patients chosen for this particular technique were all inpatients and were approached preoperatively for anesthetic evaluation. Intravenous regional anesthesia was ruled out in any patient with serious peripheral vascular disease including a history of thrombophlebitis. In addition, certain patients were

---

John J. McGlone, D.P.M., *Caylor-Nickel Clinic, Bluffton, Ind.*

excluded because of their attitude toward block anesthesia and the assumption was made that they would not tolerate the anesthetic procedure well. The procedure was explained in detail to the patients. The selected patients were given a liberal amount of preoperative medication which consisted of 75 to 100 mg of Demerol[1] and 50 to 75 mg of Vistaril.[2]

With the patient in the operating room and in the supine position, the usual vital signs were measured. An intravenous infusion was started in the upper extremity. Through this infusion a solution of 0.1% Brevital[3] was given slowly to further sedate the patient. The drug of choice used in this particular survey was Carbocaine[4] 0.5%. A two-tourniquet control system was also used along with a 21-gauge Butterfly[5] needle (Fig. 1 and 2.) Two Kidde[6] tourniquets were placed just below the knee distal to the head of the fibula and were attached to the tourniquet-inflating device (Fig. 3). A 21-gauge Butterfly needle was then placed in the dorsal vein of the operative foot as near to the site of the procedure as was possible. A small amount of Ace[7] adherent was used to facilitate retention of the tape during the surgical preparation (Fig. 4).

The leg was then elevated for 1 to 2 minutes and the area below the tourniquets was wrapped snugly with an elastic bandage from the toes distal to

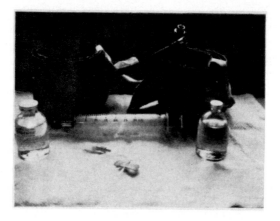

Figure 1.

[1]Winthrop Laboratories, New York, N.Y.
[2]Pfizer Laboratories, New York, N.Y.
[3]Eli Lilly & Co., Indianapolis, Ind.
[4]Winthrop Laboratories.
[5]Abbott Laboratories, Chicago, Ill.
[6]Kidde, Bloomfield, N.J.
[7]Becton, Dickinson and Co., Rutherford, N.J.

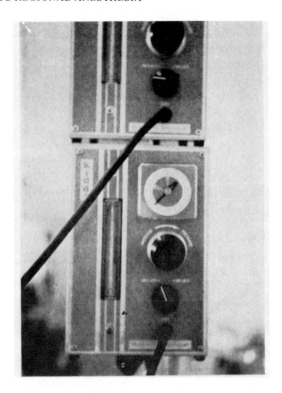

Figure 2.

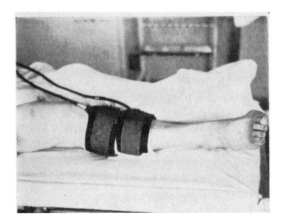

Figure 3.

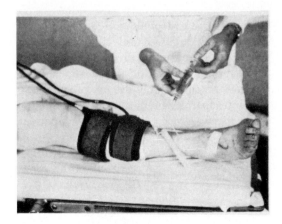

Figure 4.

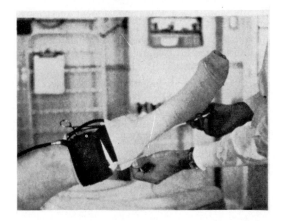

Figure 5.

the proximal tourniquet. The most proximal tourniquet was then inflated to 400 mm of mercury pressure (Fig. 5).

A 0.5% solution of Carbocaine, consisting of a total of 30 ml, was then injected via the Butterfly needle in the foot and the surgical preparation was begun (Fig. 6).

General Considerations

A vein as close to the operative site as practicable is chosen. If this is done, the onset of analgesia is more rapid and complete.

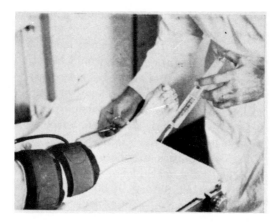

Figure 6.

The needle gauge should be as small as possible. Large bore needles are unnecessarily painful and the large hole they produce has caused difficulty because of extravasation of the anesthetic solution through the hole.

Exsanguination, prior to injection of the anesthetic solution, is essential. This prevents the dilution of the intravenous anesthetic agent by residual blood. Also, exsanguination will collapse the vascular compartment of the extremity and relative collapse of the compartment is necessary for the injected solution to be accepted. Originally, it was felt that 30 minutes should elapse before the tourniquet was released but more recent data indicate that diffusion of the anesthetic solution is complete by 15 minutes and the tourniquet may be released at this time.

Complications

1. Pain from the tourniquet usually begins after 35 to 45 minutes of ischemia. This can be alleviated by speeding up the infusion of Brevital. If this is not sufficient to control the tourniquet pain, then the pain can be alleviated by changing the site of the tourniquet pressure from proximal to distal where the anesthetic agent has perfused; thus the pressure would be on an anesthetized portion of the leg.

2. Tourniquet failure is another complication. If the tourniquet should deflate before the surgery is completed, analgesia is rapidly lost.

3. No fatalities attributable to the intravenous regional block anesthetic have been reported among 10,000 documented procedures over a span of over 60 years.

4. Generalized convulsions have occurred in intravenous regional block anesthesia necessitating treatment with barbiturates.

5. Cardiovascular reactions, consisting of hypotension, bradycardia and various arrhythmias, have been reported but have rarely necessitated treatment.

6. In this series 16% of the patients experienced incision pain. The addition of 10 ml of 0.5% Carbocaine sufficed to control the incision pain and could be added at any time after the initial injection was made.

The dose and the rate of systemic administration appeared to be by far the most important factors in adverse response to the local anesthetic agents. Virtually all the reported reactions were the result of either an excessive dose or a very rapid rate of systemic administration of the drug.

Summary

Intravenous regional block anesthesia was employed in 62 patients over a 3-year span from March 1967 through April 1970. These patients had very minimal post-anesthetic problems such as nausea and vomiting and were allowed to eat on return to their hospital room.

The toxic problems with the local anesthetics are minimal with this technique. A total of 150 mg of Carbocaine does not represent an overwhelming dose, even if it should gain immediate access to the general circulation. This complication should be rare with the technique described above.

It was anticipated that this might be a valuable outpatient procedure initially. However, at present, it would appear that because of the liberal use of preoperative and intraoperative sedatives, this technique lends itself more appropriately to inpatient surgery.

References

1. Colbern, E. C.: The Bier block for intravenous regional Anesthesia: Technique and Literature Review, *Anesth. Analg. Cleveland, 49*:935, 1970.
2. Morrison, J. T.: Intravenous local anesthesia, *Brit. J. Surg., 18*:641, 1931.
3. Holmes, C. M.: Intravenous regional analgesia, *Lancet, 1*:245, 1963.

IX. Mini Surgery vs. Open Surgery

Panel Discussion

Comments by: Clyde Shreve, Jr.

I was first introduced to osteotripsy when in the Service. While now in private practice in Ogden, Utah, I have continued to do a large amount of this work. As consultant to Hill Air Force Base, I am referred all the foot problems and especially surgical cases. I have continued to do osteotripsy on active duty, retired and dependents, as well as on a hospital and outpatient procedures basis. I think our set-up is unique, in that these patients are required to come back at periodic intervals for careful postoperative evaluation.

I object to the term "minisurgery," "burring," rasping, or even osteotripsy, when it is used to denote an inferior type of surgical approach or a less permanent one. I want to suggest to you instead, that we are dealing with one of the most important and original developments in the history of our profession. It is unparalleled, and it is not a carbon copy of approaches used by another profession. It is *all* podiatry!

I want to suggest to you that we are dealing with an approach to the treatment of foot problems that has absolutely unlimited potential. What do I mean by "potential?" The surgical correction of bunion procedures utilizing such techniques as modified Kellers, McBrides, Stones, modified Akin, Silver, and treatment of these problems with at least 75% less disability. Also, the correction of various types of heel problems, whether it be a heel spur or Haglund's disease and so on, depending upon your judgment as to whether a surgical procedure should be utilized. Once again, with a probability of at least 75% less disability. Also, the correction of all types of tarsal problems, the correction of metatarsus primus varus or plantar-deflected metatarsal ray; the complete resection of metatarsal heads, the shortening of toes; the placing of toes in any position that we choose and prefer. In other words, this is definitely not the type of rasping that most of us realize is being used in the United States today. We have found that the bone work is not the sole procedure by any means, and in many, many cases it is the soft tissue work that is most important.

Clyde Shreve, Jr., D.P.M., *Consulting Staff, Hill Air Force Base Hospital, Ogden, Utah.*

I object also to the title of this discussion: "Minisurgery versus Open Surgery." This implies that we are in some kind of "athletic event" and are competing for trophies. We are not! The very nature of the approach to our problems as we see them in our profession is to meet certain basic scientific criteria. And what are they? Such things as: will the procedure that we choose bring about a permanent correction of the patient's problem? Especially relative to conventional forms. What about function? Will it impair function? Will it improve function or will it have no effect upon function? Cosmetically – that is another important question to answer in your own mind as to what procedure to choose. What will be the cosmetic implications in this case? And then again – trauma. What effect will this procedure that we choose have upon the patient, psychologically as well as physically? It is not just a mere question of what length incision we are going to use. I think it is poor technique to try to classify approaches to foot problems in terms of lengths of incisions. Our basic object is to meet the scientific criteria. One thing I am surprised at is the great disparity in our results. As we keep in contact with each other and as we travel around different parts of the United States, I am amazed at the disparity of success in osteotripsy. I am concerned only because I realize the tremendous improvement in our results in Utah and especially as I work with my colleagues there. Gentlemen, osteotripsy is the hottest issue today and I think we all agree to that. This very discussion is an example of that.

Practically every seminar that we hold will have some topic, some discussion on osteotripsy. Often, practitioners will attend one of these seminars and afterwards take some little "nuggets" or "gems" back home with them and try to apply these in their own practice. They will have less than satisfactory results because of not realizing that we are developing certain standards by which these procedures must be performed. To follow these standards will yield amazing success. Not to follow them will often bring failure. But our colleagues will go home and try these procedures. They will have a poor result, develop a negative attitude and close their minds to this brilliant approach to the treatment of foot problems.

It is important to have an open mind and a good attitude toward any type of treatment, whatever it might be. The question is: Does it work? If it does work, we must use it. Let me give you an example of what I mean by "attitude." I attended the A.P.A. Convention two years ago in Washington, D.C. There was a panel discussion on hammertoe surgery. One of the questions posed to the panel was: "Will rasping work on digits?" A panelist stood up – and answered by saying: "No, because most digital problems are caused by toes that haven't any quality and digital length or digital position." It so happens that I agree with that comment. But there were many people there, I am sure, who went home and closed their minds to osteotripsy that very day. I am here to tell you that we have developed techniques whereby we can permanently shorten any toe that we desire, to any length that we like. We can place the toe into any position that we care to. We have had professional bracemakers working with us as assistants who have been working on digital problems of the hands.

Just because you can do a digital osteotomy – a transverse resection of bone – in less than 120 seconds from the time that skin is prepared and 84.7% of the patients do not take even aspirin; just because there is not a suture does not mean that this procedure is less effective than if the bone was resected using bone forceps, laser beam, or any other means. I submit to you the contrary.

Before I make my closing statement, I would like to say we owe a great deal to two men back East who pioneered in the development of these techniques and who continue to do so. I firmly believe, gentlemen, that the stage is set for a near-revolution in the treatment of foot problems. In conclusion; I think that we must begin and end a discussion like this by honestly asking ourselves, our colleagues (and this is the very nature of our profession): are we meeting the scientific criteria that have been set down for us? And if we are – and indeed, we are – then well and good. But if we aren't, then we must have the courage and the integrity to innovate and change.

Comments by: Earl G. Kaplan

As the last speaker said very profoundly, this is a discussion which is very difficult to present in 10 minutes. There is a lot of activity in this field, more than any place else. I have been performing foot surgery for 28 years, and during this time there have been great changes in the field of foot surgery. I don't feel that you could stand up on a platform, or any place else, and intelligently say that "This is no good," or "That is no good," because there is good and bad in all of the surgical procedures. I feel definitely that the osteotripsis has a very definite place in the field of podiatric surgery. Primarily in nail conditions, and exostosis, and uncomplicated hammer toes, it can accomplish much.

The problem is that some practitioners are increasing their scope of closed and blind surgery almost to the point where many of the claims being made are ridiculous. Statistics that they presented are valuless to the medical profession because it is done as an office procedure in the greatest number of cases (well over 90%). There is no way to judge or evaluate contraindications, e.g.: To what extent is there swelling, pain or disability, and is the result permanent. When you

Earl G. Kaplan, D.P.M., *Past President, American Podiatry Association, Detroit, Michigan.*

make a statistical study in a hospital, you test swelling by very definite testing mechanism. Testing machines are used against definite standards. There aren't any standards set for office procedures and standards are different in each office. So the statistics that are going to be presented from office surgery cannot be documented. I think that it is very unfair to a patient to perform rasping types of procedures where there are fixed hammer toe deformities and are not necessarily authentic, because the greatest amount of recurrence comes in hammer toes where there is a great amount of deformity. You can relieve prominence but the dislocation remains. Also I am against using rasping technique which is being advocated in neuroma surgery.

In metatarsal work: Right now there are several new techniques in open surgery such as removal of bases of metatarsals, and osteclasis – wedge osteotomies and other techniques which seem to produce far better results, which have definitely improved the recurrence factors. The main thing that I want to point out is that blind surgery should not replace open surgery which allows you to see everything and what is really involved. I think the most important aspect of this whole controversy is what is happening to the young men who are coming out into the field. No talk about the many complications which can develop. It is unbelievable that in our field right now it is a disgrace to take care of a nail or an excrescence palliatively. There was a newspaper article that I saw just recently about a woman who complained to a columnist that she went into a podiatrist's office to have an excrescence taken care of, which he had done for years. She was laid down without permission. The man injected the toe. He did some type of surgery. But he had no permission to do the surgery. She did not understand what was being done. She complained that she did not even have the excrescence taken care of, what she originally wanted taken care of. It was more bad publicity and greatly misunderstood. But this is the same presentation which is being done in many offices throughout the country.

We have to intellectually and honestly determine whether we are giving dollar diagnoses. This is a convenient way of making quick money and there is no doubt of it. But there is a danger of getting up on a platform and telling an audience that in 48 seconds you can remove an excrescence, and it won't ever come back again; without telling the facts of possible complications which often arise, e.g.: extensive swelling—like in sausage toes; the fact that spicules may remain in the toes; infection; recurrence; diabetes. But more especially the fact that there is a greater percentage of recurrence than in open surgery. Regeneration of bone is something that we have been seeing more than just occasionally. Hospital and pathological studies have been done regarding regeneration of bone. We find that a great deal of regeneration is found. Even after open surgery, instances where heads of proximal phalanges have been removed, we later found that complete head regeneration has taken place. If this is true in open surgery, how can you justify that in rasping procedures where portions of bone have been removed, they claim permanent removal in 96% of all cases. I think there are false statistics. I feel no real attempt has been made to really show true percentages.

Now some figures to document a few arguments:

Figure 1 is the incision of a hallux valgus procedure. The first Figure is the beginning of a hallux valgus. I just want to carry you through to the capsule part of it, and show you how large and thick a capsule is and how much destruction there can be done in going through the capsule blindly, without knowing what you can see or do.

Figure 2 shows the capsule. The exostosis below the capsule is very large. The adductor tendons which attach to the base are strong, and pull over a toe into a valgus position.

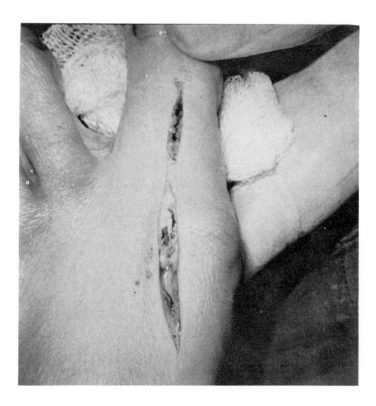

Figure 1.

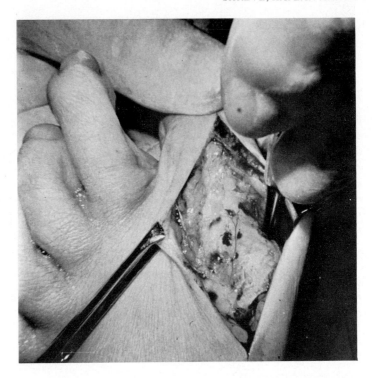

Figure 2.

Figure 3 demonstrates how we are opening up the capsule. This capsule is very, very thick. In closed surgery in which there is no knowledge of how deep you are going, and where you are going there is a tremendous amount of danger of destroying this capsule and forming scar formation with the capsule area.

Figure 4 reveals the flap of the capsule. If this capsule is destroyed, it will cause a tremendous amount of scar tissue. We have opened up a great number of these after a rasp technique has been performed and the amount of damage is tremendous. Cutting into this area after rasping is like cutting through cement. It is completely fibrosed. Correction afterward is very difficult to hold.

What I want to emphasize in this presentation is that we get the cases that fail. We see the complications when they occur. In the hands of the few experts in this field who have developed some of these techniques they are good as far as digital procedures are concerned but in the hands of other podiatrists influenced by fast talk – a great number of problems exist. The average practitioner using rasping techniques are going beyond the realm of good judgment.

Figure 5 shows how deep the soft tissue tumor lies. This is the start of the dissection of a neuroma.

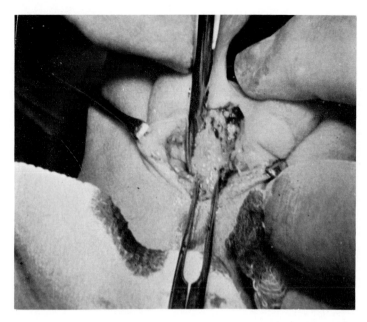

Figure 3.

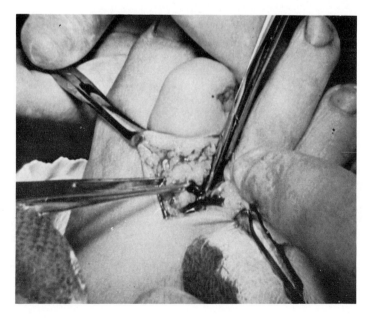

Figure 4.

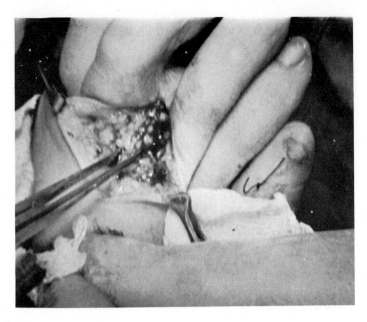

Figure 5.

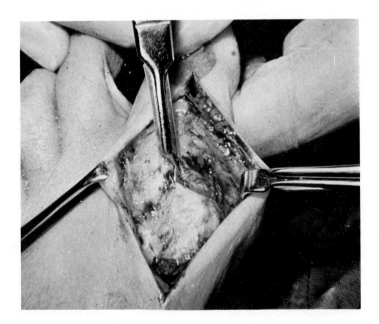

Figure 6.

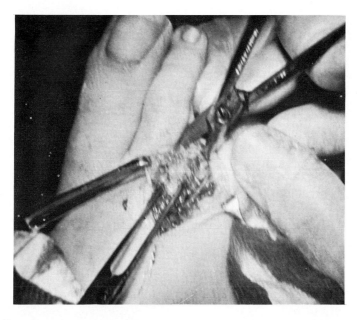

Figure 7.

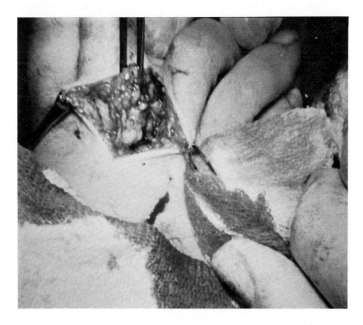

Figure 8.

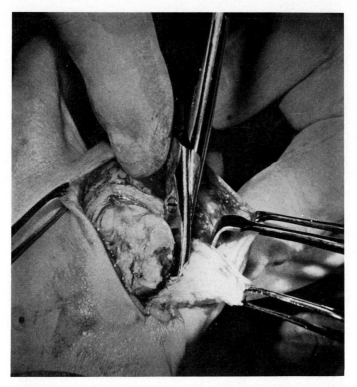

Figure 9.

In Figure 6 it is being held by an allis clamp.

In Figure 7 we are grasping it. You have to go completely under all areas and go all the way down in between the heads themselves to get the neuroma entirely out. I defy anybody to go in there and take this out with a rasping technique, which has been advocated on some of the lecture platforms.

Figure 8 shows the tumor coming out, *en toto.*

Figure 9 shows the growth itself, how big it is. If it is not removed in its entirety, you have a good chance of having it reoccur.

To sum up, if these rasping procedures are going to stand the test of time, there must be some honest evaluation done without emotion entering into it, and the fact that a lot of things are being advocated without telling about the possible contraindications that can occur as a result of the surgery or the rasping technique, is criminal. It should be told like it is — the good and the bad — and then let us judge.

Comments by: **Joseph B. Addante**

Since the news media and political controversies have made us aware of "equal time," my position on this panel is to speak with equal time for a "third" point of view, *"midi surgery."* Yes, in the battle of the mini, midi, and maxi, the midi has been a tragic failure in the fashion world; however, maybe we can champion the area of "midi" in surgical podiatry.

Since my particular interest is in the area of plantar keratoses under metatarsal heads, it is reasonable to call this the *midi part* of the foot. I prefer to approach this problem with an osteotomy or osteoclasis performed through an open incision of about 3 cm with the use of a double-action bone cutter and sutured skin closure. This is certainly not mini or stab surgery; however, neither is it maxi open surgery involving the M.P. joint such as a plantar metatarsal condylectomy would be. In keeping with biomechanical cautions of not disturbing joints, the plantar declination of the metatarsal can be altered and I believe the true classification, if we have to *"name call"* techniques would be *"a midi surgery."* It involves midi trauma, midi risk, and a midi convalescent period.

If we reflect on the purpose of this panel, we cannot avoid the fact that the mini, midi, or open maxi are not the issue involved here, but *more importantly*, what is best for the patient. I wholeheartedly endorse open-minded surgeons and "may their tribe increase." I encourage and share the desire for mini-trauma surgery and may the patients enjoy the cures of the "book of gold." Aren't we also saying that *mini-trained* surgeons are the maxi trauma? We should caution against the concept that techniques and instruments can make a surgeon.

Drills and Rasps and Techniques Do Not a Surgeon Make

We need *maxi training* with *mini professional discord* to get the maxi image of podiatric surgery. We may be mini in our thinking if we polarize on this issue. The process of evolution should be allowed to continue and yield improved techniques. The result would be better podiatric surgery for more foot-weary patients. Better foot health for more patients with reduced cost and periods of disability should be the goal: *"midi"* may be the approach.

Perhaps we don't have to open as much as we used to, and maybe the mini as a midi could prevent us overlooking what might otherwise yield less than the desired result.

With a sense of pride in podiatric contributions to human foot health, I would urge that our goal not be a "mini" or "open" one. Should we not take a

Joseph B. Addante, D.P.M. *Member, Examining Board, Massachusetts Board of Registration in Podiatry, Fitchburg, Mass.*

second look and with a "midi" reconsideration admit that the "surgical pendulum" should be ready to normalize in a midi position?

We have traveled from superficial to medical to surgical. We can now begin to enjoy the luxury of choice — mini, midi or maxi or any combinations — manual, mechanical or motorized.

With new vistas being projected, let us pick the best and be selective for those patients who *we believe were selective when they chose podiatry* to solve their foot ills. Let us be fair and give responsible thought before jumping into an attitude of over-enthusiasm toward *any* therapy.

Let's walk the midi path and keep our minds receptive to improvements and also remember that: "all change is not necessarily progress."

X. Four-Handed Podiatry: Mobilization of the Podiatric Assistant

Four-Handed Podiatry

Comments by: **Charles R. Turchin**

We must get away from the idea that only a doctor can take a heart reading. And, gentlemen, you *will* be taking heart readings. And you will be recognized. In our community, in meetings with the various carriers, we will do the work; take heart readings, circulatory readings; work that at one time was considered to be the exclusive purview of the internist. It just so happens that we, too, are doctors. We, too, know how to do this. No profession, no allied profession in medicine, has greater ability to recognize internal disorders, which manifest themselves originally on the feet, than we. Every necessary means to determine the cause should be utilized to continue to maintain this ability.

You must start thinking now of the semiprofessional group of podiatry assistants, probably some day licensed, definitely educated, and definitely reimbursed for their education; and their ability to carry on. We cannot escape this responsibility, because this can very severely affect our practice and our profession. We cannot get 28,000 podiatrists in this country by 1980. But we can get 28,000 practitioners and podiatry assistants to take care of what we otherwise would have to take care of.

I don't have to relate what happened when Medicare wisely included podiatry. I don't think I have to get a crystal ball and predict what is going to happen within the next five years when National Health Insurance becomes a reality. From our conversations with the Social Security Administration we expect five years of chaos after it has passed. Just imagine, that within 24 hours after the signing of the first National Health Insurance bill, over 100,000,000 people, who now do not subject themselves to first-class medical care, will become first-class medical patients. Look what happened in our offices when overnight 20,000,000 people became first-class medical patients. And a good portion of them podiatric patients.

So we must start now, think now, plan now, to make sure that we are prepared to receive this responsibility, and, justly so, receive this responsibility

Charles R. Turchin, D.P.M., *Retiring President, American Podiatry Association, Washington, D.C.*

as we will be given the authority. As you know, every national health insurance bill now being proposed by Congress includes podiatry.

How can this be done? By starting to train your office to work with more than just *your* two hands, to work with more than just *your* two eyes, to work with more than just *your* two ears. You must add assistants who are not podiatrists, but who are properly trained and properly educated by you to carry on duties which can be performed just as well by a nonprofessional. You must start now to build an image for your assistants, deserving of the respect and serving the desires and needs of the patients.

I know what it is to try to do everything by myself. I know how much better it is to have others do work that I used to do; and, strangely enough, they do it better. When my girl casts a foot or a fracture, it is a much better job than I have ever done. When my girl takes an x-ray, the consistency is always better. She knows her job thoroughly because she does it constantly. And I am thus freed to do highly specialized work, especially in the field of surgery. The preparation and finishing procedures of the patient are performed by the semiprofessional better than I.

So you must not fall a victim to your professional ego. Remember that you cannot operate with two hands when you need four hands, especially when the other pair of hands is quite often superior to your own in the delivery of a service! My office has six girls. When one or two of them stay home sick, I miss two or four more pairs of hands.

Above all, the professional medical podiatry assistant is a reality. Colleges are setting up, and are training and are graduating professional assistants. You must utilize them. But you must prepare your inner self also. You must prepare your physical plant. And above all, you must prepare your patient to accept and respect the professional assistant.

Comments by: Ben Hara

You and I have a difficult time hiring a podiatry assistant. The general public doesn't know the podiatry assistant even exists because the profession is not even listed as an occupation in the vocational manual. The public schools are not aware that both male and female can be trained as podiatry assistants nor does the public realize that we are seeking podiatry assistants. Consequently, there is no listing of podiatrists' assistants' curriculum in the community colleges out West.

So, what happens when you and I need podiatry assistants? We try placing an ad in the paper, contact the employment agencies, and ask staff workers to

---

Ben Hara, D.P.M., *1257 West San Bernardino Road, Covina, California* contact friends and acquaintances who may qualify. Even with this intensive search, we are required to screen between 30 to 50 people before we come up with one person who might be worth training as a podiatry assistant. Perhaps, up to now, we have relied upon the overflow of health workers or, by lucky chance, acquired suitable personnel and trained them. But the going from now on will be increasingly difficult since there is a definite shortage of competent medical personnel.

Training of the Podiatry Assistant

At present, we do not have a podiatry assistants' training program in colleges. Therefore, we have relied on the in-service training in our particular office. But there is a problem in this. How many men have the time, patience, teaching ability, plus the administrative gift, to carry out a sustained training program? What happens instead is that — in most offices — the new assistant comes in, learns the basic rudiments and does not progress much beyond that. She is left to shift for herself. Obviously, there is a sore need for college training in which assistants can receive one to two years of science and business background so that they can come to podiatry colleges, clinics, and offices to receive additional training.

Some may feel that medical and dental assistants' schools at a vocational level are sufficient for our needs. In our area, I find that schools generally do not have the high standards necessary to produce top assistants; of course, there are always exceptions when collegians enroll in such a school. In the main, there has been such a technological advance and change in the role of the podiatry assistants in the last decade, that it behooves our profession to train its own personnel in order to delegate maximally. We can no longer rely upon medicine or dentistry to do this for us. Year by year, the work of the podiatry assistant has become more complex. We must realize, as a profession, we have not begun to systematically train our podiatry assistants on a wide scale.

General medicine has a training program — both with the local colleges and cooperating hospitals. Therefore, students can train for nurses, L.V.N., nurses' aides, technicians (all categories), administrative assistants, medical records librarians, and various specialized office workers. In addition to this, they have college programs for medical social workers, chemists, physicists, engineers, librarians, medical assistants, physicians' assistants, psychologists, and pharmacists.

Dentistry started in 1913 by initiating a dental hygiene program in the office of a dentist in Brookport, Conn., who visualized the need of dental hygienists. Today, over five thousand new dental hygienists are required annually. The profession also has a college program so that they can train their dental chairside assistants, dental secretaries, and dental technicians. They have programs leading to an A.A. or A.S. in the Dental Assistant's program. Medicine and dentistry have faced the need for competent, trained personnel by initiating and maintaining such training programs.

By comparison, podiatry is way behind and unless we face the issue head-on and create a podiatry man power pool, we will continue to be confronted with the tough problem of securing competent help in our offices. With medicine and dentistry vying for one million health workers a year to replace and add to their growing service needs, we will have an even tougher time getting suitable personnel for our particular profession. It's easy enough to get help with low motivation, low intelligence, and low productivity, who are looking for 'just another job.' But podiatry needs highly-skilled assistants who can meet the technical needs of the profession and the growing demands in public and private podiatry practices.

Training the Podiatrist As Concerns
Mobilization of Podiatry Assistants

The podiatrist has multiple functions to perform simultaneously: as clinician, administrator, teacher, innovator, and P.R. man. The training of the podiatrist must take into consideration all the facets involved or the student will succeed in one or two areas only, in his general practice. But touching *all* bases is indispensable – if he is to achieve a high degree of professional excellence.

One of the ways to begin is to have a trainee assigned to undergraduates in the sophomore, junior, and senior years at the podiatry colleges. In this way, the student will be able to know – at first hand – what it means to have a podiatry assistant. He will learn how to deal with her intellectually, academically, and emotionally, and the assistant trainee will also be exposed to the needs of podiatry at a college level. This technique in the training and mobilization of the podiatry trainee-assistant is not a novel idea. Dentistry has utilized this method by assigning such personnel to the junior and senior students in dental school.

Those colleges which have a podiatry hospital can further train the podiatry assistants by assigning them to the interns and residents, when they can be under the supervision of a R.N. or holder of B.S. or M.S. versed in podiatry. In this way, they will be learning hospital protocol which will be a step in the right direction to relieve shortages of surgical technicians and nurses at various hospitals. Later on, podiatry assistants can scrub in with podiatrists at the hospitals in private practice. Only by working with patients and with podiatrists can the future podiatry assistant increase her knowledge and her skills. How well she performs will be dependent upon her motivation, and professional training. We must train our personnel to the extent that we are willing to delegate technical responsibilities to them.

The podiatry assistant is in reality the *bride* of podiatry. Only lately have we begun to recognize her as a *bride* and not as a *common-law wife!* As recently as the last decade we have begun to see assistants at our divisional, regional and national meetings. The common-law wife does not have the dignity nor the stature of the official wife: she has no pride in being what she is. We must not create such a demeaning posture for podiatry assistants. We need them sincerely and desperately in the profession. They are truly professional members of the health team.

Attracting Podiatry Assistant Trainees

We must begin to attract potential podiatry assistants from among students in high school and early college. The earlier we make the contact, the better off we are in providing specific goals for the students and claiming their allegiance to podiatry. In the same way that we have attracted podiatry students into the colleges, we must now recruit potential podiatry assistants. We should seek out and be ready to address groups of students — who are medically oriented — in high school and in colleges. We should be willing to invite those interested to visit our offices and to spend time with us. The latter must be modern and the various therapies and modalities in use there should challenge the scientific minds of students. We encourage them to go on to college so that we can utilize the body of knowledge that they will acquire and so help us eventually to upgrade our work. Two years of college work is a *must*.

The salary and benefits for podiatry assistants should be commensurate with their duties and responsibilities and should equal — or exceed — that which general industry provides. In the mind and heart of the trainees there must be the pride and prestige of being associated with a growing profession of podiatry.

Interviewing (at the office)

We should be prepared to explain podiatry through the use of brochures, podiatry college catalogs and a booklet which explains the orientation to the office and the profession. Once a student applies for training, we should be prepared with a battery of tests to determine the applicant's general intelligence, typing and spelling abilities, emotional stability to withstand stress in the profession, and determine whether the person concerned has the appearance and potential worth to be trained as a professional podiatry assistant. In addition, we should determine whether she has manual dexterity, fluidity in communication and is willing to put forth the hard work necessary to emerge as a fully fledged, competent assistant.

People who are simply looking for another job should not be accepted. Such applicants will not represent podiatry well nor will they become more productive and grow in the profession. A worthy applicant is one who will continue to study and develop her skills beyond the daily needs of the office.

We should be willing to spend anywhere — from half a day to several days — determining the suitability of applicants by giving them tests and inviting them to observe, so that *we* have an opportunity — in turn — to observe *them*. We can also provide a one-month trial of in-service program to determine the suitability of the applicant. Medicine has one month of internship without pay in the doctor's office. If we find that an applicant is very sharp and competent and gets along well with people, we can cut short the internship and offer her a full-time position.

Mobilization of the Podiatry Assistant

Pediatricians have launched a pediatric nurse-practitioner program at the University of Colorado Medical Center in Denver. These pediatric nurses will be able to handle at least 75% of the work which normally falls to the pediatrician. About 75%-80% of our work falls in a routine category. This means that we should be prepared to delegate maximally to the podiatry assistants. In order to do this, we must be sure that the duties are being delegated to trained personnel who are able to handle the work. From the patient's viewpoint, the service rendered must be identical with that of the doctor. Otherwise, the patients have every right to complain about the lack of excellence of service. Therefore, it becomes very crucial in attracting – and keeping – top podiatry personnel. In the '70s and in the '80s, we will need to change our concept radically regarding the delivery of service. The work load is going to increase daily so that what we have been accustomed to handling in two days will soon be condensed into a one day period.

With the emergence of third-party medicine and government control, we will have to demonstrate that we are indeed delivering complete and up-to-date therapy. The podiatrist's ability, together with that of his assistant – will be upgraded through a sustained training program. As the work load increases, there will be need to departmentalize into sections of physical therapy, biomechanics laboratory, medical laboratory, surgery, podopediatrics, and prophylactic podiatry. Obviously, we will become more and more involved in group practice.

In all of these areas mentioned, we, as practitioners, will be required to take the necessary basic refresher courses, we will need to be better equipped and better staffed to be able to deliver competent service. Staff must be trained to assist in all the departmentalized sections in podiatry. Their many duties will include: blood withdrawals, laboratory examinations, charge of the physical medicine department, and they will also assume an increasing role in history taking, neurological, peripheral vascular examinations and plethysmography. As geriatric patients are increasing annually, our staff must be prepared to assist maximally in homes and convalescent hospitals and know how to handle charts rapidly and accurately. Podiatry assistants can also be trained to handle part of examinations in biomechanics. It is imperative that a sustained training program be established in offices so that both podiatrists and assistants will be exposed to the reading and the discussion of medical literature. We cannot rely upon occasional lectures to close the credibility gap, nor upon periodic lectures to keep us fully alive professionally.

Pilot Program

Pilot programs must first be established in the podiatry colleges in cooperation with community colleges. Podiatrists should support the proposed program by serving on the faculty and afterwards be prepared to hire graduates of the program. The podiatry assistant trainee must be further exposed to training in foot clinics and podiatry offices throughout the United States. Once the program gains momentum, we can expand it accordingly, in terms of our actual needs. The availability of trained podiatry assistants will not just *happen.* Manpower pools must be deliberately and carefully created. Otherwise, we will always be on the "short end of the stick" and lacking in adequately trained personnel.

We live in rapidly changing times and should welcome, therefore, those changes which we see are clearly necessary in order to make our profession advance. Leadership among us must be developed in order to train suitable assistants. Other members will follow accordingly, but the followers cannot exceed the leadership in our profession.

Comments by: William Lowe

Our podiatry assistants represent us 75% of the time. Let's see if it isn't so: (1) The telephone rings. It is our assistant's smiling voice that greets them. (2) The patient comes in and it is our podiatry assistant who welcomes him. (3) Finally, on the third encounter, *I* come in and *I* treat him. And I only hope that I complement what my podiatry assistants have done for my patient already.

(4) On the fourth encounter as the patient leaves our office again, it is our podiatry assistant who cares for him. Out of these four encounters, 75% are via podiatry assistants. If they already are doing 75% of the work they are already mobilized. But our podiatry assistants are capable of doing even more if we would only let them. If there is any lack of mobilization in the office it is my fault. Podiatry assistants, yours and mine, are sharp; they are our team members — not just assistants. They represent 75% of the practice. So . . . shouldn't they be getting 75% increase in salary?

Let's follow along. For you doctors who have wives, you know your wife is not only your partner, but also an executive. She can be taking care of the baby, watching him while she is ironing. While she is ironing, she is also washing clothes in the washing machine. At the very same time, she is baking something

William Lowe, D.P.M., *Richmond, Calif.*

in the oven while she is planning the menu for tomorrow's dinner. She may even be watching television with the other eye. Doing six things at one time; already an expert on time, motion and methods. Fantastic!

It is the same with our podiatry assistants. They are versatile; they are capable. They are real executives. They, too, are able to do more than one thing at a time. Why can't the podiatry assistant be answering the telephone, and using the typewriter at the same time. Heretofore, I believe most podiatrists have been using only the two hands of their assistants. That is not enough. Four hands are still not enough! They have to be representing you with their eyes, smile, ears, their whole personality. They are the extension of *you*, the doctor. How can they extend themselves? Let's go to some of the specific items.

Let's take for example, a routine follow-up treatment. Let's see what are the specific items that go into such a treatment. Let's determine what responsibilities really could be delegated to the girls? Can it be 75% of the entire routine treatment? In the routine treatment, there is (1) preparation; then there might be the (2) excrescence; (3) the nail cutting; (4) the nail sanding; (5) the padding; (6) the charting and prescription writing. Seven items. How many of the seven items can your assistant take care of? All of them? Six? Five? Great! Let's say five. Good. But how many people here will delegate these tasks to an assistant?

Making use of our podiatry assistant's talent once again, how about adhesive strapping follow-ups? I'll name a few more items: (1) Removing the previous tape. (2) Examination of patient. (3) Preparation for taping, such as cleansing the skin surface and applying the adherent. (4) Cutting out the tape. (5) The actual application. (6) And the charting. Six items. Out of these six, most of us are doing all of them, aren't we? How many of these six items can be delegated to our podiatry assistants? Four? Splendid! If even three, we're still winners, aren't we?

What about treatment of warts? Again, let's itemize its treatment. (1) Removing the previous padding. (2) Debridement. (3) Application of medication. (4) Application of the padding. (5) Charting the record. Five items. Again, how many of these can be delegated to our podiatry assistants? Four? Excellent! That is what we do in our office. Debridement only.

What about preoperative procedures in the office? Let's itemize some of these. (1) Preoperative examination. (2) The pedal pulses. (3) Blood pressure. (4) Oscillometric indexes. (5) Recording the findings such as hair growth, temperature, skin lesions. The laboratory workup, such as urinalysis, obtaining hemoglobin, and venapuncture for blood sugar. Aren't these items our assistants can be doing? Train them. Delegate.

After the surgery, our assistants can apply the post-operative bandaging. They can give the entire post-operative instructions and chart the surgical recordings. On the patient's return visit, again, our podiatry assistants are able to take care of the redressing, suture removal and post-operative x-rays.

Our gals are capable and they can do it all, if only you, the doctor, will only teach and delegate them. You *have* to delegate, because you are going to be seeing two and three times as many patients in order to serve the health needs of our country. And for those of you who are seeing too many patients already, it means more time for your golf, coming to meetings, learning more.

From our brief presentation about these few items, the program title, "Four-Handed Podiatry Assistants" might well be changed. The word "assistant" is not adequate enough. These gals are our team members. They are on the executive level; they represent 75% of your practice. Shouldn't they also get a 75% increase in salary?

Panel Discussion

DR. TURCHIN: We want to mention at the outset, "the Podiatrist's Creed." This Creed pledges us to deliver quality service in the best manner that we can. It is inconceivable that we could be seeing this number of patients without having four hands, or six hands, or even eight or sixteen pairs of hands to be sure that we deliver this quality service.

The podiatrist entrusts much of the work to the assistant. It is teamwork. Four hand functioning together.

Charting is done by the assistant.

DR. LOWE: Once in awhile, when we are rushing in and out and the gal is charting, I have to whisper to her, "P.N." "P.N." I have to call for the initials which stand for "patient's name" because I have forgotten the patient's name in rushing in and out. And this is the little clue to the gal when I say, "P.N." This is the clue for her to bring up the patient's name in the conversation so that I recognize it.

DR. HARA: We must also remember that the doctor's handwriting is no longer a handwriting but a temperature chart. And so the girl's writing would be far better. To the left of the chart upon each entry in our office we are entering both the doctor's name and the assistant's name so that we know who charted it.

DR. LOWE: In prescription writing, both Dr. Hara and I have a photography book with the celluloid slots, just about the size of a prescription blank. We would write the prescription or type it in as we would do normally in the office. On the back of the prescription blank, because it is clear on both sides, is a picture of the medication, the manufacturer's name, very briefly, the U.S.P. name, the usual dosage, and the contraindications. So the prescription writing can be done by our assistants.

Assistants are valuable in padding or palpating for a lesion. If you would train your assistants in the basics — whether it is in biomechanics or anatomy —

to be very specific in the location of lesions and the size of lesions, you will find that it will save you much time and confusion later on.

DR LOWE: Surgical redressing can be done by the podiatry assistant.

DR. HARA: It is very imperative that you have training sessions in bandaging. We spend much time in bandaging. We set aside one hour per week on Thursdays devoted completely to training without any interruptions — not even the phones are answered because the exchange picks it up. Because bandaging is not simply covering over our own errors, it is very essential that we apply it correctly, and that it looks professional. Because we will be judged by what goes out of our office, we will be judged on our ability and our professionalism. So this is a walking advertisement, not to mention the therapy.

We found that the assistants can handle much of the prophylactic care. Unfortunately, with the present statutes, the role of the podiatry assistant is not defined. We hope that sufficient latitude can be given to them legislatively so that they will not need to function in many of the grey areas as they do in the present time. For example, if this were a wart case, all I would do is trim the top a little bit and debride it. To the trained assistant, I would say, "Put an operture shield and some salisacom," and the trained assistant can handle it from there.

DR. LOWE: There is no reason why, once you have ordered the proper tests, your assistant cannot do the venipuncture withdrawal and complete packing and mailing. Some of our offices have their own setup of procedures, including urinalysis, blood sugar, and hemoglobin determination.

DR. HARA: It is amazing what the podiatry assistants can do for you. We have entitled it, "Four-Handed Podiatry," but the mind and the orderliness that they bring into the office is incredible.

DR. LOWE: Placing a thermometer in their mouth, this is what you do to stop a patient from talking.

DR. HARA: Yes, always carry a thermometer in your breast pocket. It really does the job. You know, it reminds me of these two ladies who were horribly crippled. They had arthritis of their temporal mandibular joint and they couldn't move their mouths. They were horribly crippled!

You know, if we had to do all of this work that the wonderful podiatry assistants are doing, we would have to block off an hour or an hour and a half of our time. As it is, all that we do for, say, an H.D. fifth where we are doing proximal arthroplasty is to allow six to ten minutes of our time. All other parts — the preliminaries, and the after work, is taken care of by our assistant. They even write our prescriptions for us. It is a very, very wonderful way to practice.

DR. TURCHIN: I would like to bring up a very important point. We all think of podiatry assistants as female. There is no reason under the sun why a podiatry assistant can't be a man with training in the Medical Corps of the Army or Navy or Air Force. You have some educated men who also want to get into a semiprofessional skill and they also can be utilized.

DR. HARA: We may attract those, too. Hopefully, if we get the male podiatry assistants I think we would have a greater stability as far as turnover of personnel goes.

DR. TURCHIN: I agree with that. I would also like to make another point. This is most important in my own personal office. My girls are not allowed to take any history whatsoever, but only allowed to go ahead and take recordings and put it down. For instance, I have right now three associates in my office: podiatrists who are never allowed to ask of a new patient this question: "What is your main complaint?" I am very strong on that point. It is very important for patient rapport that wherever possible the doctor walk in, recognize and, if possible, put his hand on that complaint because I think the greatest amount of referrals that I get is from the patient who leaves and tells their friends, "I walked into the doctor's office and the doctor immediately knew what was wrong with me!" That is one of the most important things. I cannot go for the idea of the girl asking the patient: "What is your name? Address? What is your main complaint? How about this? How about your heart? How about this?" This I believe is a doctor's prerogative. It goes back many years with me. When a man came into my office, I said, "What is your trouble?" He said: "I came here for you to find out and tell me."

The podiatry assistants that we need today has multiple roles. She is (1) a surgical technician, she is (2) a lab technician, she is (3) a physical therapist, and as one of the speakers has said, she is (4) also a diplomat, she is (5) a communications expert. She is many things in one. And therefore in order to be able to delegate successfully we continue to look for high caliber personnel. In the profession we can't always have work done by rote. Judgment is necessary. And so we are seeking personnel who can exercise professional judgment.

DR. TURCHIN: I think both Dr. Hara and Dr. Lowe would both agree with me, when I say, that it is amazing how many patients will telephone me before they come into the office and want to know if a certain girl is there that day. The girls actually build up a following for themselves because of the sincerity in their work that they transmit to the patient.

DR. LOWE: We try not to have the patient follow one particular assistant. We try to make a team effort out of it. We try to avoid these particular attachments.

DR. TURCHIN: We try to avoid it, but sometimes you can't. Patients have individual likes and dislikes. Especially in my office.

DR. HARA: You know, in our office, the patients do ask for certain podiatry assistants or you can see by body language how happy they are to have certain assistants. I am praying right now that some day they are going to call on me to come in and see them.

DR. TURCHIN: We find that true in our office, too.

DR. HARA: It would be irreversible damage that could be committed by an uninspired, uninformed, untrained assistant to give you the wrong medication, wrong dosage. We want to have the kind of assistant that you and I would be happy to have minister to us.

DR. LOWE: In our office, after the medication is withdrawn, a sterile syringe is placed in contact with the empty bottle. This is to let me know which bottle this was withdrawn from. The sterile syringe is placed in contact with the bottle from which the medicine was withdrawn. This is in direct contact.

DR. HARA: It is important that when you make your contacts with your Joint Commission accredited hospital or even non-Joint Commission hospitals, that you train your personnel well; that they do not break sterile technique. You realize that with the R.N.'s and with the surgical technicians, if any break in sterile technique occurs they are going to be called upon to make an accounting. Thus far, we have not had one assistant criticized for that reason to the point where the hospital has asked us not to send that particular assistant. We have been very careful and very successful. On the other hand, we had one incident recently where the orthopedic surgeon brought in his assistant, and the Executive Council at the hospital went into session and asked the orthopedic surgeon not to bring his assistant because of repeated breach of sterile technique.

The assistant should be able to recognize promptly and correctly all instruments of the hospital as well. They should be professional in every sense of the word — their movements, their language, their self-confidence.

DR. LOWE: There is a circulating nurse who records and charts the procedure right away so that before the patient leaves, the insurance forms are sent out.

DR. HARA: We have had assistants who looking over our shoulder have in the past recorded complete surgical reports. I have just been amazed how quickly they do this. They look over our shoulder, and they say, "Oh, yes, a 5.5 centimeter dorso-lateral longitudinal incision was made at the first metatarso-phalangeal joint." They are writing down the report as they see it. It is amazing how well you can train them.

DR. HARA: The technique of injection, the recommended way. We used to give it high, fairly high, now we are giving it a little lower so that we can rapidly apply a tourniquet above the site of the injection. The same thing holds true for giving injections in the buttocks. If the patient goes into reaction, where are you going to apply the tourniquet?

DR. LOWE: I save that for myself instead of giving it to an assistant to do.

DR. TURCHIN: The stockroom is rather important, too. A lot of us don't see the necessity for a properly arranged, properly controlled area for materials used in the office. And quite often we find ourselves in an emergency. This is an important job for a podiatry assistant. She should properly arrange it so that it will properly work.

DR. HARA: They are so dedicated and such sweet spirits that I say again: Tap their talent early in life. Commit them for a lifetime for the betterment of our profession.

DR. LOWE: Our girls are also very talented in the ortho lab. The complete fabrications of orthotics are done by our assistants. It is a lot less expensive than sending the work out.

DR. HARA: As I was looking over the curriculum that Dr. Richard Lanham gave me, he had a curriculum inclusion of "Biomechanics" which I think is a very important part of the college curriculum.

MODERATOR ROSENFELD: We have a few questions from the audience which I think are important enough to introduce at this time. They are directed to all three of the speakers: What is a fair salary for (1) a beginner; (2) one that is trained; (3) benefits?

DR. TURCHIN: I think it is rather hard to pick a specific salary as Ben pointed out in his talk. There is no classification for podiatry assistants. If you look at classification in any vocational book, they give you a range of salaries that has not occurred. And, of course, salary would also vary according to the basic training prior to their entry into your associateship. You certainly cannot pay a girl who has graduated from high school the same basic salary as a girl who has acquired a baccalaureate degree in science at college. So you can't give a specific answer. Regarding benefits, my girls get health insurance, sick leave, the same as any other competitive business. There is a business side to the practice. We do know what the average salaries are in our community and we start them off accordingly. Each of you knows what it is in your community, too.

In my office we have a kitchen in which they cook their own lunches.

DR. LOWE: To answer the question, I like to give them specific numbers. As Dr. Turchin mentioned, it varies in different areas. I come from a little cabbage patch in Richmond, California, and we are in competition with industry there, so the very lowest we have been starting out with for a girl with no experience at all – nothing, no how, no where – the very lowest, lowest, lowest is $350.00. We increase that $25.00 per month. If the girl is somewhat better, we start her at $450.00. Our high is $600.00 per month. This includes overtime and fringe benefits. Our fringe benefits include sick leave, paid vacation, and seminar time. If they come to a seminar or meeting, the time is given to them along with room and board. Employees who have been with us longer than one year are invited, with their husbands, to attend the seminar with us – for example, at Disneyland in our area. These are our fringe benefits.

DR. HARA: I think that the salaries in doctors' offices will vary according to the geographical regions. We are thinking of anywhere from $400.00 to $600.00 as a salary. And, Bill, I notice that in your office, after about a year, you give the employee who has been with you one year a salary of $500.00 for competent personnel.

DR. LOWE: Right! If they are good, they belong with you. If they are no good, they should be discharged after the second or third month.

MODERATOR ROSENFELD: Here are a couple of questions that are almost the same, directed at you, Ben. Do you have any material for testing your prospective podiatry assistant? Do you have any organized forms or tests for selecting an assistant, and is it possible to obtain the same?

DR. HARA: I believe that each podiatrist's office is an extension of that podiatrist's personality and needs. I recommend that you start out with a simple manual listing the various needs. There are several books out. Teddy Clarke's book, The Ohio College Book of The Ohio Podiatry Association is out and I understand that Bill was the editor. These can be wonderfully incorporated along with the management textbooks such as that of Dr. Egerter. You can utilize all of them. My favorite is Cotton. Cotton really says something to me.

DR. TURCHIN: I make a point in my office to never hire a girl until she is also interviewed by my Number One Girl in the office, because the Number One Girl is the one who will have to train the new girl. She gives her the basic training, and there should not be a personality clash at that point.

I'd also like to bring out that if you are near a college or a university, which has a testing psychology set up, they will sell you certain questionnaires which you may give to the girls to see if they qualify to enter into a certain type of work. Dr. Selby of Washington, D. C. uses this testing service and has been successful in getting girls who are interested in the medical care professions. And it is available in various parts of this country.

DR. LOWE: Dr. Turchin has mentioned "university." This brings to mind recruiting the podiatry assistant. Our office is near the University of California at Berkeley. This is where we try to obtain our podiatry assistants. The husband, for example, is going to school for four years or, maybe, two years of graduate school. We want the wives. They are young, sharp, and they know that they have to support a husband through college. This is where we try to obtain them, and I am sure that you can do the same thing.

DR. HARA: May I also suggest for your testing that you use a Minnesota multiphasic Personality Inventory. This is done by your local psychologist, and he will quickly send you back a personality profile, to especially determine whether this young lady is emotionally suited to your particular work.

Seriously, we are also using the computer testing. Those who are going into keypunch and computer programs have tests which you can get at your local store. They have a number of abstract tests – the kind where you have your particular drawing of diagrams, inverted, and so forth, to be matched. I think that it is very wonderful to be able to test their intelligence and ability in abstract thinking. Manual dexterity tests are also given – gloving, using oxygen, giving oxygen, using scissors, and using the Jack sander – just to quickly test their manual dexterity.

MODERATOR ROSENFELD: Here are a couple more questions for you, Bill. First, how long does it take you to train a new office assistant?

DR. TURCHIN: I find that in my office, we don't expect a new assistant, or even a podiatrist, to know too much before six months.

DR. HARA: It is very unusual when you have a girl who turns out at three months. She is a jewel. Hang on to her. If she'll let you.

DR. TURCHIN: That's the best type to keep on after three months.

MODERATOR ROSENFELD: The other question is: How do you train your office assistants to make presentations to patients in the office?

DR. TURCHIN: I don't permit it.

DR. HARA: Very seriously, we have training sessions where we pose situations that are quite common and we have group sessions where we hear each other out. One is the patient and the other is the one who is communicating with the patient. We throw the question out. This is a situation and we see how they handle it. Unless they are given this responsibility to verbalize, to communicate, they will never really develop the communication abilities. So just like the preceptees and the interns who are coming in, they don't know how to properly communicate yet. And so we help both the preceptees and the assistants with a training session in communications.

MODERATOR ROSENFELD: The grey area, I presume, is the delegating of the palliative care of the patient by the assistant. If this trend should catch on in podiatry, are we not alerting the public in medicine that nonprofessionals and illegal persons can do the job? Where will we get our surgeries from then?

DR. TURCHIN: Of course the entire trend in podiatry assistants in this country is not to give them diagnostic authority or singular right to work, similar to an R.N., who does a great deal of work – injections, x-rays, and quite often, first aid work. Yet she is not permitted to do it unless there is a physician present. Whether or not the trend will continue in medicine, they are trying to train assistants who will diagnose and set fractures in hospitals under the jurisdiction, of course, of the Department of Orthopedics or whatever department. I can see that there is a possibility that podiatry assistants will be cutting callouses and doing work of that sort. I can see a slight trend toward that. Because there is just not enough manpower. However, the complicated work would be left to the doctor. At the same time, they will not be allowed to treat unless a doctor is present.

DR. HARA: May I answer that grey area, in regard to venipuncture, and so forth. It is the area that would normally fall into the technician's area. This is what we are referring to when we speak of "grey areas." Many of these areas are not really defined. Even the removal of sutures is a technician's area, or realm, perhaps, in the mind of progressive practitioners. We must be very, very careful on one point. We should underline this. And that is this: delegate, yes; but relinquish, never. You can delegate but never do you relinquish direct supervision.

XI. The William J. Stickel Awards Selected Papers

A Study to Determine the Relative Absorbability and Wicking Effect of Certain Major Sock Materials on Perspiration of the Human Foot

James A. Davis

Acknowledgment

No research paper would be complete without giving credit to those who helped in its completion.

I am indebted to Anthony Goyena, Ph.D., of Kayser-Roth Hosiery Company, for his patience and able assistance in the preparation of photographic and statistical techniques.

My thanks go also to head football coach S. S. (Red) Wilson, his assistant coaches, trainers, and the football players of Elon College, Elon, North Carolina, for their complete cooperation during these series of experiments.

Introduction

For many years, podiatrists and dermatologists have been searching for a sock that would absorb perspiration and move the moisture away from the foot.

Many materials and mixtures have been suggested with varied and generally unsatisfactory results.

More recently with the advent of the synthetic materials, there is a wider choice, making the podiatrist or skin specialist confused to know which sock material to recommend for the average healthy foot, not to mention the pathologic hyperhydrotic one.

Moisture and humidity will not allow the human wastes of the skin to evaporate,[1] creating more heat in hot weather. It would seem likely that a moist foot would also have a greater likelihood for frostbite in sub-freezing temperature.

James A. Davis, D.P.M., *Burlington, North Carolina.*

The rate of evaporation of water is influenced inversely by the degree to which the environmental atmosphere is already saturated with moisture.[2] Sweat which is not evaporated but simply drips from the skin, of course, does not increase heat loss. For this reason the sweating mechanism is badly crippled when the relative humidity is high.

The amount of perspiration normally secreted depends upon the temperature, relative humidity, and the muscular activity of the individual. At moderate temperature, evaporation keeps pace with secretion, and no actual drops of sweat form. This is known as *insensible perspiration* and is obviously the optimum condition for the skin of the foot.

Therefore, maintaining the foot in as nearly perfect an environment as possible insofar as socks are concerned would (a) reduce urea deposits on skin, (b) sodium chloride and other salts, (c) in turn hold pH in a normal range, and (d) lean toward an equalized perspiration index.

Certainly, a moist foot does not heal well surgically, and a wet skin is more susceptible to fungal and bacterial infiltration.

Winter sports enthusiasts, hunters, and military men are aware of the importance of dry feet. A sock that allows less moisture to accumulate next to the skin would lessen frostbite and also would be more comfortable to the wearer during warmer periods.

Purpose

Theoretically, if there is more moisture on the outer surface of a sock, there should conversely be less inside on the surface of the foot, thus a healthier sock for all climates.

The purpose of this study is to show differences in the "wicking" effect in certain sock materials, demonstrating that the sock with the greater "wicking" ability is a more comfortable, healthier sock because of the drawing away of moisture from the foot surface to the outside of the socks during vigorous exercise periods.

Method

To determine the relative absorbency and "wicking" effect in certain sock materials, the method used for the purpose of this study was as follows:

A. To measure the amount of moisture on the foot before and after exercise, sheets of blotting paper were used which had been impregnated with cobalt chloride.

B. Socks of varying compositions were used as follows:

    1. Sock #1313, composed of 100% Banlon* nylon (See Fig. 1).

---

*Trademark Registered Joseph Bancroft & Son Co.

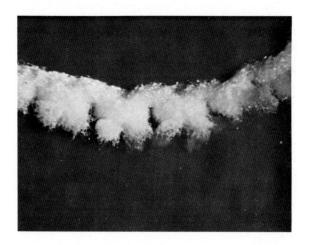

Figure 1.

2. Sock #1800, composed of 65% Orlon† acrylic, 25% cotton, 10% nylon (See Fig. 2).
3. Sock #3000, composed of 32% cotton, 33% wool, 35% nylon (See Fig. 3).
4. Sock #1275, composed of 68% wook and 32% nylon (See Fig. 4).

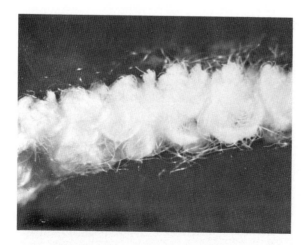

Figure 2.

†Trademark Registered E. I. du Pont de Nemours & Company

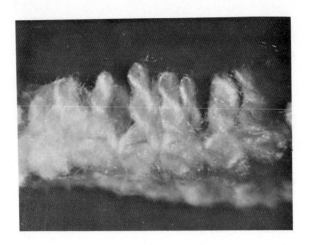

Figure 3.

5. Sock #5284, composed of 65% Orlon, 25% cotton, 10% nylon (See Fig. 5).
6. Sock #1250, composed of 80% cotton and 20% nylon (See Fig. 6).

After each imprint was taken, color photographs were made.

In addition to the photography of the cobalt-impregnated paper, pH paper was adhered to each foot of the tested subjects, and also the skin temperature was recorded through a small hole in the sock before and after exercise periods.

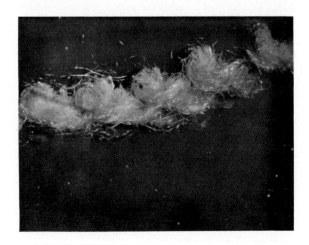

Figure 4.

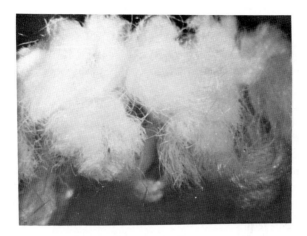

Figure 5.

Subjects

Twenty players were selected for each test from a college football squad‡ and divided into groups.

The groups were selected primarily because of their excellent general health and normal foot structure. Their feet were examined and only those considered to be normal in sweat excretion were used in the experiments.

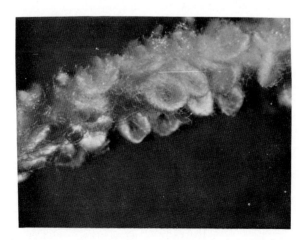

Figure 6.

‡Elon College, Elon, N.C., S. S. Wilson, head football coach.

Procedure

A. Strips of pH tape were adhered to each player's feet just posterior to the web spaces.
B. Socks of different compositions were given to each subject for each foot and recorded.
C. The skin temperature was taken on each foot at the plantar surface, at the web area through a small hole in the sock, before practice and recorded.
D. The time was recorded after the players had put on their football shoes to begin their practice session. Temperature and humidity were also recorded.
E. After the practice session of approximately two hours, the players were brought in, their shoes removed, and the skin temperature immediately taken through the hole in the socks. At no time did their feet touch the floor surface.
F. The players then stood on the cobalt sheets, with their socks still on, for fifteen seconds. Immediately upon stepping off the sheets, a color photograph was taken (See Fig. 7A).

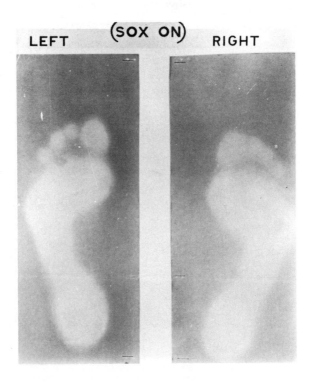

Figure 7A.

G. Their socks were then removed and the same procedure was followed by the players stepping on fresh sheets of cobalt paper to check the *surface* moisture of the bare skin (See Fig. 7B).

Sock #3000 composed of 32% cotton, 33% wool and 35% nylon measured superior to all tested socks.

The second best sock #1800, composed of 65% Orlon, 25% cotton, and 10% nylon, was constructed with a heavier cushion on the plantar portion of the sock. It was assumed that this sock might possibly surpass the others due to its unique knitting.* The tests showed differently however.

A second series of tests was completed using only styles #3000 and #5284. Style #3000 had been used for military purposes. Style #5284, used extensively as a ski-sock, had almost three times the weight of ordinary socks. In this test each sock was weighed before the football practice and was recorded in grams. After the practice period, these same socks were weighed and compared for weight increase.

LEFT (BARE) RIGHT

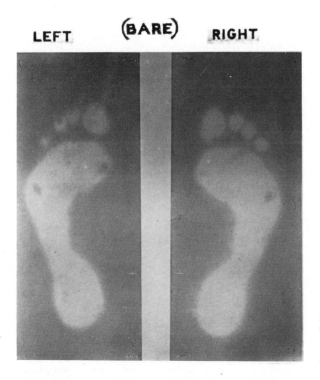

Figure 7B.

---

*"Birdwick", Kayser-Roth Hosiery Company, Inc.

Tables 1 and 2 show the weights of the socks, the weight of perspiration absorbed in grams, and the percentage of moisture contained in each sock after practice session.

Results

A. Sock #1250, 80% cotton and 20% nylon, was eliminated in first test for the following reasons:
   1. Absorbed little water.
   2. Showed little temperature control.
   3. Showed heavy residue of perspiration on the foot.
   4. Wrinkled badly during exercise.
B. Sock #1313, 100% Banlon, was eliminated from further testing because:
   1. Foot surface was extremely moist after exercise.
   2. Was not durable.
   3. Wrinkled badly during exercise.
C. Sock #1275, 68% wool and 32% nylon:
   1. Showed better results in perspiration absorption tests.
   2. Wrinkled badly during exercise scrimmage and rolled down into shoes, and was poorly accepted by players for this reason.
D. Sock #1800, a combination of 65% Orlon, 25% cotton, and 10% nylon, showed good results.
   1. Did not roll down into shoes.
   2. Maintained fairly constant temperature in cool temperature, but heated the foot in higher temperature periods.

TABLE 1. Temperature, pH and Weight Gain.
Style 3000 — Military Sock

Player	Temp. Before Exercise	Temp. After Exercise	Weight Sock Grams	Weight Sock After Exercise	Weight Gain Grams	Percent Gain	pH
1XXX	84.5	89.5	27.471	30.305	2.834	10.30	5.5
2XXX	81.5	86.0	27.020	29.585	2.565	9.47	6,0
3XXX	95.0	76.0	26.805	28.625	1.820	6.80	6.0
4XXX	80.0	75.0	27.095	27.605	0.510	1.89	6.5*
5XXX	78.5	81.0	27.148	19.165	2.017	7.43	6.0
6XXX	88.5	79.5	26.679	27.695	1.016	3.81	6.5
7XXX	95.0	92.0	27.258	29.840	2.582	9.45	6.5
8XXX	92.0	93.5	27.842	31.050	3.208	11.55	7.0
9XXX	77.0	77.5	26.500	27.150	0.650	2.45	7.5*
10XXX	83.5	80.0	27.348	28.860	2.512	9.20	7.5*
Ave.	85.6	83.0	27.117	28.988	1.971	7.27	

*Taped Ankles

TABLE 2. Temperature, pH and Weight Gain.
Style 5284 — "Birdwick" Ski-sock

Player	Temp. Before Exercise	Temp. After Exercise	Weight Sock Grams	Weight Sock After Exercise	Weight Gain Grams	Percent Gain	pH
1XXX	84.0	87.5	64.378	68.205	3.827	5.94	5.5
2XXX	84.0	90.0	66.457	72.695	6.238	9.40	6.0
3XXX	94.0	75.0	66.153	67.165	1.012	1.73	6.0
4XXX	80.5	82.5	65.425	67.062	1.637	2.50	7.5*
5XXX	84.0	86.5	64.405	67.340	2.935	4.54	6.0
6XXX	85.5	81.5	64.540	65.810	1.270	1.97	6.0
7XXX	90.0	92.0	65.900	68.352	2.452	3.72	7.5
8XXX	91.0	92.0	65.440	70.260	4.820	7.38	7.5*
9XXX	77.0	85.0	68.070	69.195	1.125	1.65	7.5*
10XXX	83.0	87.0	67.349	73.512	6.163	9.17	7.0*
Ave.	85.3	85.9	65.812	68.960	3.148	4.77	

*Taped Ankles

3. Absorbed considerable moisture and moved it fairly well from foot to outer sock surface.

E. Sock #3000 composed of 33% wool, 32% cotton and 35% nylon, gave top performance in all categories.

1. Better temperature control.
2. More moisture on outer surface of sock.

TABLE 3. Comparative Color Differential Between
#3000 and #5284 Ski-sock

Player	Type Sox		With Sox		Without Sox		Color Differential
	Left	Right	Left	Right	Left	Right	
1XX	5284	3000		+	+		+2 (3000)
2XX	5284	3000		+	0	0	+1 (3000)
3XX	5284	3000		+		+	- 1 (3000)
4XX	5284	3999		+	+		+2 (3000)
5XX	5284	3000		+	+		+2 (3000)
6XX	5284	3000		+	+		+2 (3000)
7XX	3000	5284	+			+	+2 (3000)
8XX	3000	5284	+			+	+2 (3000)
9XX	3000	5284	+			+	+2 (3000)
10XX	3000	5284	+			+	+2 (3000)

+ = Any color change from opposite foot
0 = No color change from opposite foot

3. Less moisture residue on foot surface.
4. Comfortable to wear with little rolling down or wrinkling.
5. Good player acceptance.

Discussion

Of all the tested socks, those containing the combination of 33% wool, 32% cotton and 35% nylon kept the feet drier and cooler in normal to very high humidity and temperature (60° to 90° range.)

As was predicted, the foot remained drier when the outer surface of the sock showed more moisture.

It would seem from these experiments that the wool, cotton, and nylon are most desirable socks for average to high temperatures and average to high humidity.

The pH factor seemed to have no bearing in these tests and varied according to each individual tested. However, one strange factor did arise: In every case if a player had his feet and ankles strapped before scrimmage, the pH rose from a pH of 5.5-6.5 up to a pH of 7.5-8.5 after two hours of practice and scrimmage. Those players *not strapped* showed little or no change in pH.

The second sock tested that showed superb qualities for athletic wear was the thicker ski-sock composed of 65% Orlon, 25% cotton, and 10% nylon knitted in the "Birdwick"* pattern. (See Fig. 5.) This sock, though two and one-hald times the thickness and weight of any other sock tested, absorbed numerically (by weight) more moisture; still it contained only half as much moisture percentage-wise as any other sock tested.

This ski-sock, though very thick, was considered by most of the athletes tested to be the most comfortable. Although the thinner socks tested kept the feet *drier and cooler during hotter temperatures, the athletes still preferred the thicker sock for comfort.*

Conclusions

This study of determining the relative absorbability of certain sock materials has brought out some interesting data.

A. For moderate temperatures to very hot, humid temperature, a sock containing 33% wool, 32% cotton, and 35% nylon (similar to military sock) kept the foot cooler and drier during rigorous exercise.

B. For extremely cold conditions, a much thicker sock with 65% Orlon, 25% cotton, and 10% nylon knitted in the "Birdwick"* pattern proved to be exceptionally comfortable, gave less wrinkles, caused less blisters, and was most accepted for general comfort by the athletes tested.

---

*Kayser-Roth Hosiery Company, Inc.

C. The pH does not change significantly after rigorous exercise except with those athletes having had ankles strapped with adhesive.

D. During very hot weather, the temperature of the foot tends to equal the outside temperature. In some cases the temperature may even *decrease* during extensive exercise (tending to equal the air temperature) even when enclosed in regulation football shoes and athletic socks.

Summary

A. Unique testing methods have been used to determine the relative dryness of the foot in contrast to the relative moisture retained in socks after extensive exercise.

B. pH of the skin before and after exercise was not significant except in the subjects who had had their ankles strapped; for in each case, the pH went to higher alkaline readings. Further testing in this area should prove interesting.

References

1. Best, Charles, and Taylor, Norman: *Physiological Basis of Medical Practice*, Baltimore, 1945.
2. Kleiner, Israel S.: *Human Biochemistry*, St. Louis: The C. V. Mosby Company, 1945.

The Damaging Effects of a Disaligned Musculoskeletal System

Charles L. Jones

Acknowledgements

The roentgenographic studies of the pelvis and knees were performed by the Osteopathic X-ray Laboratory and the American Hospital of Chicago. I would like to thank Gwen Hammar and Bruce R. Abraham for their kind assistance.

Introduction

Diseases due to abnormal posture are not recognized as such; however, it is readily accepted that abnormal posture can bring about a serious disturbance in function. A prolonged disturbance in function may lead to pathologic changes which are recognized as a definite morbid process. The two diseases that are most obviously affected by disalignment of joints are rheumatoid arthritis and osteoarthritis. The cause of rheumatoid arthritis is unknown but the overall comfort and well being of the patient are greatly influenced and improved by maintaining proper joint alignment. The disalignment of involved joints increases mechanical irritation, which promotes further destruction, inhibits function, and increases pain. Osteoarthritis is the direct result of mechanical irritation of involved joints. Lack of lubrication[1,19] and/or faulty alignment increases wear and tear on joints, thereby causing degenerative changes. Osteophytic proliferations in the form of spurs, lips and bridges, and articular margin incongruity are the cardinal signs of a disaligned or imbalanced joint.

Effecting proper postural alignment of the lower extremities is overwhelmingly neglected. Practitioners have failed to place in proper perspective the fact that uncorrected postural disalignment of the feet and superstructure can cause relevant maladaptive changes. The functional adaptation of the musculoskeletal system to the changes produces pathomechanical problems and morbidity that

---

Charles L. Jones, D.P.M., F.A.C.F.S., *Chicago, Illinois.*

are irreconcilable with normal stance, gait, and posture. The development of hallux abducto valgus as a result of functional adaptation of the first metatarsophalangeal joint to an underlying foot problem is all too common a condition. The insidious development of a chronically puffy-edematous ankle in women, from years of wearing shoes which did not offer stability to the foot and ankle, is another simple but very common morbid state. This gives evidence to the soft tissue changes that can occur around a joint subjected to very brief periodic disalignments over a long period of time. Disabling low back pain caused by a discrepancy in leg length is a classic condition of a postural problem.

The purpose of this paper is to establish the significance of the fundamental involvement of clinically unapparent disaligned musculoskeletal systems in the development of and the resultant pain from osteoarthritis, lumbosacral problems, sciatica, discogenic disease and certain static foot problems. The necessity for having weight-bearing roentgenographic studies performed on feet, ankles, knees, pelvis, and lumbar spine will be made apparent in order to evaluate adequately the relationship of posturally disaligned feet with the superstructure, and vice versa. The corroboration of the interrelationship between certain disease states and postural disalignments will be upheld, in that the early damaging effects of the disalignments were reversible and/or the patients experienced distinct relief from the pain caused by the acute pathology, when proper balance and symmetry were restored to the foot or to the extremity. This should give insight into the necessity for effecting postural alignment to ameliorate immediate problems, and, equally important, to prevent future morbidity.

In Consideration of the Foot

Representative pedal conditions that can cause postural disalignment of feet are calcaneovalgus, calcaneovarus, forefoot varus, forefoot valgus, etc. It is these primary conditions that can give rise to secondary conditions such as hallux abducto valgus, digiti quinti varus and flexion deformity of the digits.

A brief discussion on a very common roentgenographic finding will serve as evidence in discussing the maladaptive changes resulting from an underlying foot problem. An increase in thickness of the second metatarsal has been recognized as a good example of static transformation of bone. This is acknowledged as the normal response of a bone that is forced to intermittently bear more weight or stress than was initially intended. A short first metatarsal in the so-called Morton's syndrome or a hypermobile first ray will cause the second metatarsal to be forced to withstand more body weight (Fig. 1a and b). The compensatory hypertrophy usually is sufficient to prevent the metatarsal from having a stress fracture; however, under extreme physical stress upon the metatarsal, there can be a spontaneous dislocation of the respective digit (Fig. 2).

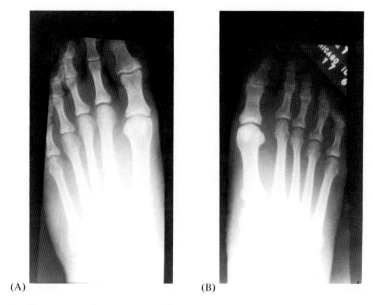

(A) (B)

Fig. 1a. Hypertrophied second metatarsal associated with a short first metatarsal. **b.** Hypertrophied second metatarsal associated with a hypermobile first ray evidenced by diastasis of the first ray from the second.

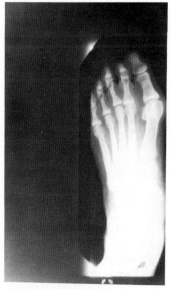

Fig. 2. Spontaneous dislocation of second digit. Note hypertrophied second metatarsal and diastasis between first and second rays.

The result from pathomechanical stress at the level of the first metatarso-phalangeal joint is less picturesque roentgenographically but more damaging, and may be instrumental in the development of hallux abducto valgus. This is readily observed clinically when the anterior aspect of a hypermobile first metatarsal is forced into a dorsally abducted position during stance and pre-propulsive phases of gait, which causes the hallux to be forced into an abducted valgus position. When the metatarsal head is round and there is considerable external pressure on the hallux, the ability of the musculature to stabilize the hallux is greatly depreciated, developing the deformity more rapidly (Fig. 3 and b). If the metatarsal head is square in shape, the tremendous force that the articulation is being subjected to is evidenced in "squaring" of the joint margins, lipping or spur formation around the margins, or a flattening of the articular surfaces (Fig. 4).

These secondary problems could be avoided by controlling the underlying hypermobility of the first metatarsal or accommodating for the short first. It is understood that if the hypermobility is a result of an underlying foot problem, then treatment of such would alleviate the problem. Thus the importance of early diagnosis and treatment of posturally disaligned feet is apparent. Other analogies could be presented but this should suffice to make it evident that secondary maladaptive changes due to underlying postural problems could have been avoided.

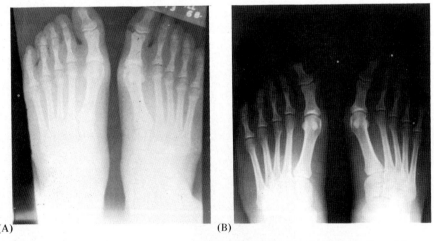

(A)   (B)

Fig. 3a. Early hallux abducto valgus development in a 14-year-old girl. Note the epiphyses are not closed; the second metatarsals are hypertrophied; there is diastasis between the first ray and the second, there is eburnation along the medial aspect of the head of the first metatarsal; and there is lateral displacement of the sesamoids. **b.** Same patient three years later. Patient has been wearing foot orthotics to control postural disalignment. Notice there is no further development of hallux abducto valgus.

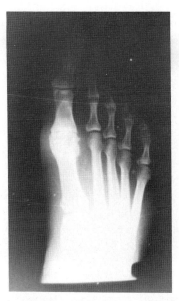

Fig. 4. There is flattening of articular surface, medial and lateral lipping of articular margins, decreased joint space associated with diastasis of first ray and hypertrophied second and third metatarsals.

In Consideration of the Ankle

The ankle joint allows motion in the sagittal plane and adjusts the line of gravity in standing. The joint that adjusts the line of gravity from side to side is the subtalar joint, and allows motion in the frontal plane. The transverse axis of a normal ankle joint in an upright standing position is perfectly horizontal. Therefore, any condition which would affect the side-to-side positional range of motion of the subtalar joint, or would cause a deflection of the normal line of gravity from the superstructure, would force the axis of the tibiotalar joint to deflect from the horizontal (Fig. 7a). This is readily observed in a foot that has calcaneovalgus. The head of the talus courses more medially and plantarly than normal, causing the leg to be rotated inwardly on the foot. The foot, in turn, assumes an outwardly rotated position on the leg. With such a pathomechanic situation, there is increased wear and tear on the involved joints and an earlier evidence of joint degeneration (Fig. 5a and b). 1

In Consideration of the Knee

In a roentgenogram of a normal knee joint in the standing upright position, the transverse axis is perfectly horizontal. Any change in the internal tension stress on the transverse axis would cause increased wear and tear on the medial

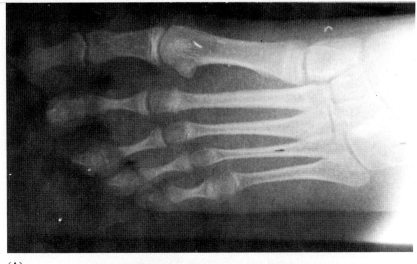

(A)

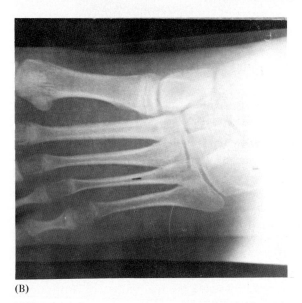

(B)

Fig. 5a. 11-year-old girl with untreated calcaneovalgus. Notice the diastasis between the first ray and the second metatarsal and the hypertrophied second metatarsal. b. Close-up of midtarsal area reveals squaring of joint margins with early marginal beaking of first cuneiform. These findings are indicative of excessive wear and tear on the joints and are the early signs of osteoarthritis.

Comment: Early treatment is mandatory to prevent further joint changes and subsequent degenerative arthritis and, equally important, to prevent secondary static foot conditions.

or lateral condylar tables and associated surrounding soft tissue (Fig. 6). Steindler[16] quotes Micularz, a German investigator, as reporting that "the weight-supporting line through the axis of the femur strikes the knee joint with only slight deviation in 87.5%, with slight medial deviation in 12.5%. A deviation amounting to more than 2.5 cm from the midline must be considered as pathological." The internal tension stress can be decidedly influenced by axial rotation of the tibia, as found in torsion problems, or by a foot problem which causes a distortion of the ankle joint, resulting in an upward retrogressive imbalance of the knee. If the relationship of the femoral head to the acetabulum varies excessively from the normal, and/or if the stabilizing musculature and ligamentous structures are out of equilibrium, the knee joint could be subjected to definite damaging mechanical stress.

The pain and discomfort that patients experience from such patho-mechanical stresses on the feet, ankles, and knees come to the awareness of the practitioner in the complaints termed as tired, painful feet, aching legs, arthritis, etc. Of course, the hallmark of pedal postural imbalance is callosities. These supposed innocuous dermal excrescences are often the first sign of the damaging

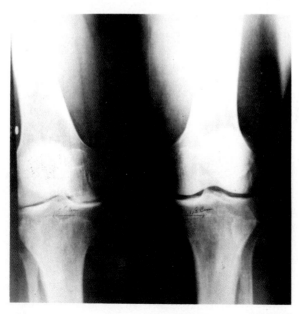

Fig. 6. 34-year-old male with one half of an inch shortage on the right side. There is a marked shift to the left of the midheel line. The medial edge of the left tibial articular surface is carried 5.5 cm to the left of that line and the right one only 1.8 cm to the right of that line. The right articular surface is perfectly horizontal whereas the left is noticeably deflected. There is considerably less joint space revealed in the left knee than in the right.

effects taking place from an unapparent disalignment. If such conditions are treated perfunctorily there will usually be a future of remissions and exacerbations with the gradual worsening of the condition and/or symptoms. In final analysis the agonizing chronicity of the problem is judged to be a matter of fact.

The importance of postural balance and symmetry can be unequivocally confirmed by the distinct relief of symptoms that patients experience when their disaligned feet are maintained in a more normal attitude. The retrogressive influence of properly aligned feet is clinically substantiated in the unsolicited comments of patients with the relief of pain and discomfort in the knees and hips. This should sustain the use of appropriate foot orthotics from the pediatric through the geriatric years, if necessary, to prevent maladaptive changes or to alleviate the disease entity.

In Consideration of the Trunk

The roentgenographic study of the pelvis, hip joints, and lumbar spine is imperative to ascertain their relationship to the trunk as well as to the lower extremities. An additional benefit will be the readily available evidence of the secondary changes that are resulting from discrepancy in leg length, and pelvis and spinal distortions.

The ascertainment of a vivid and thoroughly practical roentgenographic study is most important. Whether an x-ray laboratory or a practitioner performs the study, it is imperative that certain factors are standardized. The patient must be standing erect, have feet symmetrically placed, knees straight, and the midheel line superimposed on the center line of the roentgenograph. Antero-posterior roentgenograms should be taken of the pelvis, lumbar spine, and dorsal spine.[3,4,7,9] This technique has more value than the scan-o-gram of the lower extremities for limb inequality. The scan-o-gram involves the actual mensuration of the length of the osseous components. Leg length discrepancy is determined by the difference in measurements of the contralateral limbs. The first technique allows for a more practical study of deviations or causes of asymmetry, such as obliquity or rotation of the pelvis, developmental anomalies, acquired deformities, and sacral disalignments. The relationship between such deviations and actual leg length discrepancy can be established. It is interesting to note that in the author's studies many patients evidenced no difference in contralateral mensurations, but had a very definite leg length discrepancy due to other causes. Several patients were found to have a difference in actual osseous length patterns but evidenced a shortage on the supposed longer side. Thus the importance of considering other factors becomes readily apparent in determining leg shortages.

There are certain factors that must be noted in studying roentgenograms. The roentgenographic interpretation is made by using the iliac crests, the horizontal sacral top, femoral head tops, and the symphysis pubis as landmarks and points of reference in determining their relationship to the body planes. Consideration must be given to the shift towards or away from the midheel line of the various components of the skeletal system. The symmetry of the body is evidenced by the contralateral parts being equidistant from the midheel line and the various osseous landmarks being equidistant from the floor[7,3]. (Fig. 7b and c).

Denslow and Chace[3] report that the apparent importance of a discrepancy in the heights of the femoral heads is that the asymmetry produces an unlevel base of support for the pelvis and vertebral column. This malalignment can produce relevant maladaptive changes as we will discuss later. Rotation of the pelvis and tilting of the sacrum are greatly influenced and enhanced by leg length discrepancy. Equally important, they can be the cause of such. Singularly or concomitantly they have a pathomechanical effect on the lumbar spine. An analysis of these entities and their effect is appropriate.

Pelvic rotation is not well reported in the literature. Denslow and Chace[3] reported that pelvic rotation was considered present "... where two of the following three findings were observed: (1) a deviation of the symphysis pubis laterally from a line through the median sacral crest or the natal creases, (2) a narrowing of the obturator foramen, or (3) an apparent enlargement of the ischial spine." They also reported that pelvic rotation usually occurred contralateral to the short limb side. Such a shortage would cause some degree of lateral flexion and rotation of the lumbar spine. Denslow and Chace[3] state that Steindler described these disalignments as " ... being convex side rotation (lateral flexion to one side and rotation to the opposite side) and concave side rotation (lateral flexion and rotation to the same side)."

Some causes are not evidenced roentgenographically. Leg length discrepancy may be a result of tightness of the hip shruggers on one side, weakness of the lateral abdominal and quadratus lumborum muscles on the opposite side, and contracture of hip abductors or adductors.[2] Any angular deformity of the knee causes secondary limb shortening. Ambulatory rotational extremity patterns, unilateral rotational extremity patterns, and unilateral foot problems could also cause leg length discrepancy.

The sacrum can be given the same analogy as the femoral heads in regard to being a base of support. The sacrum supports the spine. An intrinsic sacral tilt due to a disalignment at the unions of the contralateral sides of the pelvis, or due to an anomaly such as sacralization of the transverse processes of the fifth lumbar vertebrae can affect the balance of the spine and especially the lumbosacral region[8,10,15,18] (Fig. 7c and 8b). A tilt caused by extrinsic factors such as a shortage has a comparable effect.

Hagen[7] states "... that sacral base tilt occurred to the same side as the short leg in 72% of the subjects as adults and 66% of the childhood subjects ..." in his

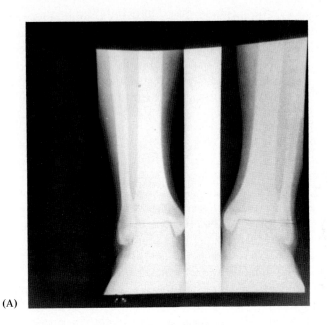

(A)

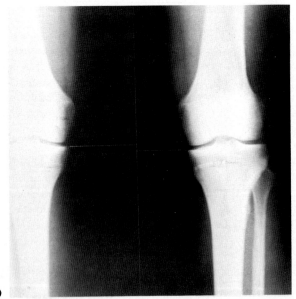

(B)

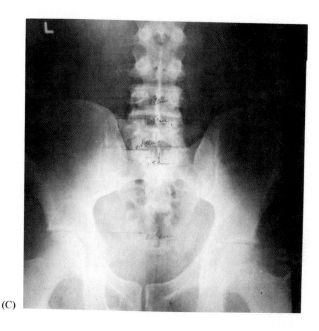

(C)

Fig. 7a. 31-year-old male complained of low back pain in the morning upon arising and generalized aching legs upon long term standing. Patient gave no complaint regarding his feet. Feet appeared normally aligned except for slight calcaneovalgus on the right foot. The left ankle mortise is perfectly horizontal whereas the right is deflected. **b.** The edge of the medial surface of the left tibia measures 0.7 cm higher from the floor than does the similar point on the opposite side. There is a shift to the left at the knees. The medial margin of the left tibial articular surface is carried 7.9 cm to the left of the midheel-line, and the similar point on the right tibia is carried 5.9 cm to the right of the midheel-line. **c.** The left femoral top measures 0.65 cm higher from the floor than the right. The left iliac crest measures 0.7 cm higher from the floor than the right. The fifth lumbar vertebra is atypical in that it developed a hypertrophied transverse process on the left – bat-wing deformity – which appears to articulate with the top of the sacrum on the left side and thus actually becomes the weight-bearing sacral top. Hence measurements will be of two types – the true sacrum and the weight-bearing sacrum. The right half of the horizontal surface of the true sacrum measures 0.4 cm higher from the floor than the left half. The left half of the weight-bearing sacrum measures 0.5 cm higher from the floor than the right half. The midpoint of the first sacral segment is carried 1.5 cm to the right of the midheel-line whereas the symphysis is carried well over that line. The lumbar area forms a mild group curve convex on the left – indicating marked stress in the weight-bearing mechanism.

Comment: A scan-o-gram of the lower extremities of the same patient reveals an apparent shortening of the length of the left femur of approximately 1 cm as compared to the length of the right femur. The two roentgenographic studies were performed by different laboratories. It is evident that the first study revealed more information. Patient was rendered asymptomatic by applying one quarter of an inch lift to the right shoe to compensate for the pelvic and spinal imbalance rather than to accommodate for the short left femur.

report of continuing roentgenographic study of school children. Thus, here again, unilateral leg length discrepancy was found to cause flexion disalignments.

When the base of support for the spine is out of balance, there, in fact, lies the basis for increased mechanical stress at the lumbosacral region and the cause for pathomechanical compensatory disalignment of the vertebrae. The lateral flexion deformity and the related rotation of the vertebrae that is usually associated with unilateral leg length discrepancy are possibly the underlying factors that initiate the pathogenesis of low back problems. James[8] reports that one of the most common types of painful scoliosis is primary idiopathic lumbar scoliosis. It seldom, if ever, requires correction or fusion, but frequently becomes painful at the onset of middle age. He also states that "osteoarthritis was evident on roentgenographic examination in 26 cases out of 33, and disc degeneration in 17." Since James[8] termed the lumbar scoliosis "idiopathic," I believe he failed to recognize the influence of an imbalanced base of support for the lumbar spine in the development of the scoliosis. The findings in lumbar scoliosis is in keeping with the flexion deformity and rotated vertebrae as found in static lateral imbalances. The wear and tear of normal mechanical stress on the intervertebral joints can be increased if the joints function pathomechanically. For an example, a part that is slightly axially rotated out of alignment would be more susceptible to the effects of torsion than if it was not.

Farlan, et al,[5] summarized in part their findings on the effects of torsion on the lumbar intervertebral joints in regard to producing disc degeneration as follows:

It was found that injury to the joint could be produced by slowly applied rotation in amounts within the range of normal lumbar movement.

Disc rupture, induced experimentally by torsion, produced changes similar to those seen in naturally occurring disc degeneration; suggesting that both changes were the result of the same conservative mechanism.

It is postulated that in vivo, disc degeneration is due to imposed torsional strains rather than to compression loads. Since the joints between the articular processes stabilize the intervertebral joint against torsion, it is suggested that any impairment of the function of the joints between the articular processes may result in a higher risk of disc degeneration.

This author would hypothesize that in many cases of acute back problems it is the presence of a static lateral pelvic imbalance with the associated flexion deformity and rotated vertebrae that predisposes the individual to the crisis. The influence of torsion in normal "unguarded" movements is sufficient when carried through a predisposed area of pathomechanical abnormality to cause acute pathology.

The corroboration of the interrelationship between static lateral pelvic imbalance and acute back problems is found, in that many patients have had complete relief from pain from previously diagnosed conditions such as osteoarthritis, sciatica, lumbosacral sprain, and disc herniation after lift therapy has been instituted (Fig. 8a, b and c).

A review of the literature evidenced a concensus that there is no one individual that has a completely symmetrical skeletal system. With this fact in mind and with the many factors to consider when analyzing a skeletal system for disalignment, it appears to be a monumental task to clinically diagnose the cause of the disalignment. Considering both statements together, the heretofore obvious unconcern over clinically unapparent disaligned musculoskeletal systems is appreciated. However, with the adept use of roentgenographic studies, disalignments are more easily recognized. The import of detecting clinically unapparent disalignments lies in the fact that no two individuals will compensate, or are capable of compensating, for their postural inequities the same way. Minor deviations can cause major distress to certain individuals in contradistinction to the major defects for which the individual compensates very well.

Early recognition is mandatory to prevent future problems. Detection of postural disalignments should be stressed in childhood. Pearson[1][2] conducted roentgenographic study of rural school children from 1947 through 1952. The objective in 1947 was: "To determine what relationships, if any, existed between the mechanical faults of children, which usually are not associated with symptoms of musculoskeletal dysfunction, and similar faults in adults, who do experience symptoms referable to the musculoskeletal system." In his published report, he stated that it appeared that asymptomatic children possessed the same types of vertebral and pelvic roentgenographic patterns as adults who experience symptoms of musculoskeletal dysfunction.

Hagen[7] also conducted a roentgenographic survey on children from 6 years of age and extended on into adulthood of 19 years to 24 years. He reported the following:

Forty-four per cent of the cases reviewed showed very close resemblance between adult and child films. An additional 10% showed generally the same vertebral patterns with minor changes. Twelve per cent of cases, although they did not resemble the original films, could be seen to have developed from curves present at an early age. Sixty six per cent of cases could be recognized in the adult films when compared with childhood films. Equally significant is the fact that thirty four per cent of cases did not present adult morphologic patterns similar to those of children.

Based on the findings of Pearson and Hagen, remedial therapy in childhood is of the utmost importance to prevent the continuance or progressive worsening of the static lateral imbalance and impending compensatory maladaptive changes. The importance of lift therapy is brought out by Klein, Ridler and Lowman[9] who performed a clinical and statistical study over a three-year period and found that idiopathic static lateral pelvis, leg, and spinal column discrepancies of elementary school boys could be treated most successfully with heel lift therapy. They reported that 61.7% had correctional gains to complete bilateral pelvic symmetry, standing and sitting. It was equally important that they noted that

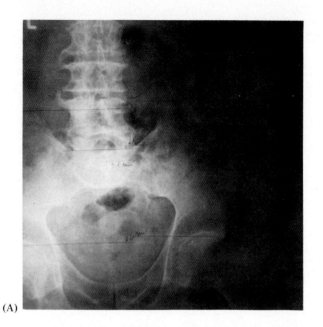

(A)

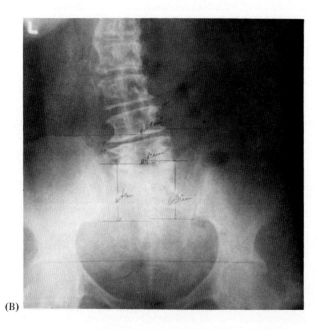

(B)

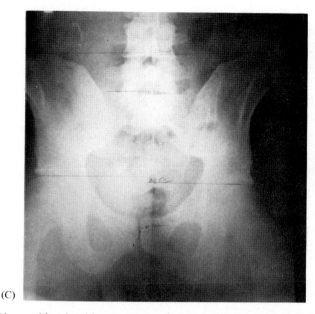

(C)

Fig. 8a. 64-year-old male with one quarter of an inch shortage on the left side. Patient had suffered with sciatic pain in right leg for past several years. Patient was told he had generalized arthritis and that nothing could be done. The right femoral top, the right half of the horizontal sacrum top, and the right iliac crest each measures respectively 0.6 cm, 0.4 cm, and 0.8 cm higher from the floor than do similar points on the opposite side. The midpoint of the first sacral segment and the symphysis are carried to the left of the midheel-line 3.4 cm and 2.7 cm respectively. The lumbar area of the spine forms a marked scoliotic type group curve convex on the left. Also lumbar vertebrae 2, 3, and 4 reveal marginal lipping laterally on the left side. The left psoas muscle reveals a very slight density increase. The pain in right leg was alleviated with lift therapy. **b.** 71-year-old woman with sacroiliac joint distortion, "sacral tilt," causing marked pelvic and spinal imbalance distortion. Patient suffered from chronic back pain. The femoral tops measure equidistant from the floor. The right half of the horizontal sacrum top measures 0.4 cm higher from the floor than the left. The right iliac crest measures 0.6 cm higher from the floor than the left. The midpoint of the first sacral segment is carried well over the midheel-line, whereas the symphysis is carried only 0.5 cm to the left of that line. The lumbar spine in combination with an unrevealed portion of the lower thoracic area forms an acutely-angled scoliotic type group curve–convex on the left with vertebral bodies rotated to the left. The body of L. 3, L. 4 and L. 5 reveals moderate degree marginal lipping. She was made relatively asymptomatic with lift therapy to compensate for sacral tilt. **c.** 22-year-old male with one quarter of an inch shortage on right side. Previous diagnosis was of a slipped disc. Patient experienced remissions and exacerbations over a five-year period. The left femoral top; the left half of the horizontal sacrum top; and the left iliac crest each measures respectively 0.65 cm, 0.3 cm, and 0.2 cm higher from the floor than do similar points on the opposite side. The midpoint of the first sacral segment is carried well over the midheel-line, whereas the symphysis is shifted 1.2 cm to the left of that line. The lumbar spine tends to form a slight group curve convex on the left–a stress mechanisms related to the short lower extremity mechanics. Patient made asymptomatic with heel lift.

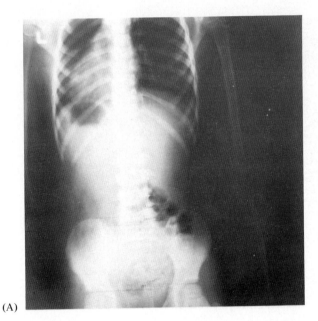

(A)

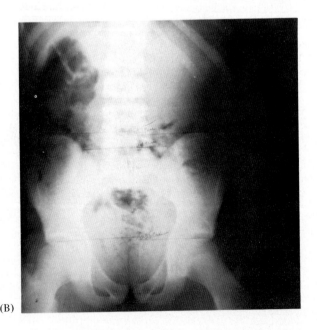

(B)

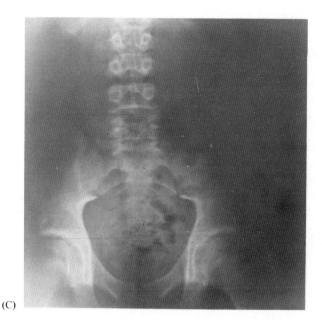

(C)

Fig. 9a. 4-year-old girl with one quarter of an inch shortage on left side. The right femoral top; the right half of the horizontal sacrum top; and the right iliac crest each measures respectively 0.5 cm, 0.4 cm, and 0.6 cm higher from the floor than do similar points on the right side. The midpoint of the first sacral segment and the symphysis measure 1.1 cm and 1.0 cm to the left of the midheel-line. The lumbar spine in conjunction with the lower 7-8 thoracic segments forms a mild "C" curve convex on the left—with the apex of the curve at the level of the first lumbar vertebrae. **b.** 9 12-year-old boy with one quarter of an inch shortage on right side. The lumbar spine forms a well-defined convex group curve on the left. The left femoral top; the left half of the horizontal sacral top; and the left iliac crest each measures respectively 0.35 cm, 0.1 cm, and 0.5 cm higher from the floor than do similar points on the opposite side. The midpoint of the first sacral segment and the symphysis are carried to the left of the midheel-line 0.7 cm and 1.2 cm respectively. The lumbar spine forms a well-defined group curve convex on the left with vertebral bodies rotated to the left and indications are that the thoracic area forms a group curve convex on the right—thus creating an "S" curve for the total spine. The lumbar group curve actually is a third stage accommodation distortion for the primary short lower extremity on the right. **c.** Roentgenographic pictures of 9b one year later after one quarter of an inch lift was applied to right extremity. Compare findings. With the patient standing – with shoes on and a 0.7 cm elevation on the right – the right femoral top measures 0.2 cm higher from the floor than the left. The right half of the horizontal sacrum top measures 0.2 cm higher from the floor than the left. The iliac crests measure equidistant from the floor. The midpoint of the first sacral segment is carried well over the midheel-line, whereas the symphysis is carried 0.7 cm to the right of that line. The lumbar spine in combination with a portion of the thoracic area forms a group curve convex on the left.

the findings in the control groups of their study did not have spontaneous correction during the growing years.

White[17] states that discrepancies up to three inches can be compensated for without symptoms of back strain but that any discrepancy over an inch and a half requires therapy. Most practitioners maintain that leg length discrepancies of one inch or less are insignificant. However, all of this author's lift therapy has been administered to patients who had clinically unapparent disaligned skeletal system of one half inch or less. Creating balance and symmetry relieved the pain of many patients which had been previously diagnosed as being that from sciatica, diskogenic disease, lumbosacral sprain. Dramatic relief was obtained in those patients suffering from osteoarthritis.

In the author's investigation and studies, there has been a certain degree of idiopathic lumbar scoliosis deformity associated with all unilateral leg length discrepancies. In cases of young people, secondary curves were beginning to be produced to compensate for the primary lumbar curves[6] at a very early age (Fig. 9a, b and c). This has special significance in children. If a child has a static lateral imbalance, and from this disalignment comes flexion deformity and rotated vertebral bodies — which is in essence lumbar scoliosis — is it not safe to hypothesize that the pathomechanical situation can be the precursor of osteoarthritis, muscle spasm and pain, possible neurological problems, and diskogenic disease in later life? The latter are the acute pathological entities that are recognized as disease states. They represent the culmination of maladaptive changes that had their beginning before ossification maturation, and were passed on to the mature skeleton as precursors for the insidious development of a disease state. Years pass before the pathomechanical problems give rise to acute pathology. People in the middle age and older are usually the sufferers of such postural problems. If the functional adaptation of the disaligned skeletal systems has not been too destructive, therapy aimed at bringing the musculoskeletal system back into balance and symmetry will ameliorate acute symptoms of pain and discomfort. If the damaging effects are too extensive, then more radical or sophisticated measures must be utilized to resolve the patient's problem, if possible.

Summary

Clinically unapparent disaligned musculoskeletal systems are fundamentally involved with the development of, and the resultant pain from, osteoarthritis, lumbosacral problems, sciatica, certain static foot conditions, and diskogenic disease. The insidious maladaptive changes that occur from an asymmetrically aligned skeletal system go unrecognized until a specific morbid entity presents itself. Usually therapy is erroneously directed at the acute pathology rather than at the underlying pathomechanical state. The corroboration of the interrelationship between certain disease states and postural disalignments, is the reversibility of the damaging effects of the disalignment, and/or the distinct relief of pain from the disease state, experienced by patients when proper balance and symmetry are restored with appropriate orthotics and lifts.

References

1. Barnett, C. H.: Wear and Tear in Joints: An experimental study. *J Bone & Joint Surg, 38-B*: 567-575, May, 1956.
2. Blount, W. P.: Unequal leg length, American Academy of Orthopaedic Surgeons Instructional Course Lectures, vol. XVII, Ann Arbor: J. W. Edwards, 1960, p. 218.
3. Denslow, J. S., and Chace, J. A.: Mechanical stresses in the human lumbar spine and pelvis. *J Am Osteop A, 61*:705-712, May, 1962.
4. Eaton, J. M.: The effect of staples on epiphysial growth. *J Am Osteop A, 60*:969-972, August, 1961.
5. Farfan, H. R., Cossette, J. W., Robertson, G. H., Wells, R. U., and Krauss, H.: The Effects of Torsion on the Lumbar Intervertebral Joints. The Role of Torsion in the Production of Disc Degeneration. *J Bone & Joint Surg, 52-A*:468-497, April, 1970.
6. Ferguson, A. B.: Roentgen interpretations and decisions in scoliosis, American Academy of Orthopaedic Surgeons Instructional Course Lectures, vol. VII, Ann Arbor: J. W. Ewards, p. 160, 1950.
7. Hagen, D. P.: A continuing roentgenographic study of rural school children over a 15 year period. *J Am Osteop A, 63*:546-557, February, 1964.
8. James, J. I. P.: Two Curve Patterns in Idiopathic Structural Scoliosis. *J Bone & Joint Surg, 33-B*:339-406, August, 1951.
9. Klein, K. K., Redler, I., Lowman, C. L.: Asymmetrics of growth in the pelvis and legs of children. A clinical and statistical study 1964-1967. *J Am Osteop A, 68*:153-156, October, 1968.
10. Larson, N. J.: Sacroiliac and postural changes from anatomic short lower extremity. *J Am Osteop A, 40*:88-89, October, 1940.
11. Patriquin, D. A.: Lift therapy. A study of results. *J Am Osteop A, 63*:850-854, May, 1964.
12. Pearson, W. M.: Early and high incidence of mechanical faults. *J Am Osteop A, 61*:18-23, May, 1954.
13. Redler, I.: Clinical significance of minor inequalities in leg length. *New Orleans Med Surg J, 104*:308-312, February, 1952.
14. Rubacky, G. E.: Claw Toes. An Early Sign of Lumbar Diskogenic Disease. *JAMA, 214*:375, October 12, 1970.
15. Steindler, A.: The Pathomechanics of the Sacrolumbar Junction, American Academy of Orthopaedic Surgeons Instructional Course Lectures, vol. XII, Ann Arbor: J. W. Edwards, p. 117, 1955.
16. Steindler, A.: Kinesiology of the Human Body, Springfield, Illinois: Charles C Thomas, Publisher, 1955, p. 331.
17. White, J. W.: Leg length discrepancies, American Academy of Orthopaedic Surgeons Instructional Course Lectures, vol. VI, Ann Arbor: J. W. Edwards, p. 201, 1949.
18. Willis, T. A.: Abnormal anatomy of the lumbosacral region with reference to low back pain, American Academy of Orthopaedic Surgeons Instructional Course Lectures, vol. V, Ann Arbor: J. W. Edwards, p. 276, 1948.
19. Wright, Verna: Lubrication and Wear in Joints, London: Sector Publishing Limited, Publisher, J. B. Lippincott Co., American Distributor, 1969.

Abducted and Adducted Gait Problems

Brian A. Rothbart

During the normal ontogenetic development of the individual, remarkable growth changes are occurring within the lower limb, the majority of which take place in the first three years of life. This growth is represented by two separate and quite distinct processes: (1) There are torsional changes occurring in the shaft of the femur and tibia on the transverse plane, and (2) there are positional changes occurring within the hip joint on the transverse plane. Both take place concurrently, and if either becomes aberrant, faulty foot mechanics are manifested as the child grows older.

Clinically we divide the lower limb into two parts: an upper and lower segment. The former comprises the femur and hip joint, the latter encompasses the tibia and knee joint.

Our purpose is to familiarize the reader with the normal ontogenetic transverse plane development of the lower limb. Armed with this information, the clinician can readily recognize and intelligently treat dysplasias resulting from aberrant growth patterns, clinically manifested as excessive abducted or adducted gaits. It will be demonstrated that one's success or failure rate in treatment depends on the practitioner's ability to recognize whether he is dealing with a torsional or positional deformity and from what level the problem arises.

The first section of this paper discusses the normal growth patterns seen in the upper segment of the lower limb. This ontogenetic development can be disturbed in one of four ways. The positional or torsional growth can become excessive causing an internal femoral position or external femoral torsion, respectively; or the growth of the limb can be stunted, producing either an external femoral position or an internal femoral torsion.

Brian A. Rothbart, D.P.M., *San Diego, California*

In the latter section of the paper, we focus our attention to the normal ontogenetic growth of the lower segment. The transverse plane dysplasias resulting from abnormal development are discussed along with courses of treatment.

When an adult femur is placed on a flat plane so that the posterior condyles lie flush on that plane, by sighting up the shaft on the transverse plane, one notes an angular relationship between the head and neck of the femur with respect to its posterior condyles (Fig. 1). That is, there is a torque present within the shaft of the femur and we can see that this torsion is located somewhere in the upper part of the femur. The angle formed from this torque varies normally between 8-12 degrees in the adult. However, a neonatal exhibits a torsional angle of approximately 30 degrees (Fig. 2). This angle reduces as the child undergoes his normal growth, and is considered to have reached its adult value by the child's sixth year of life. Hence we find a 20 degree torque change in the normal development of the femur (Fig. 3).

In the adult we define this 8-12 degree torsional angle as antetorsion. We do so because it is an anterior torsion of the head and neck of the femur compared to its distal condyles. Any angle less than the adult value produces a structural relationship referred to as retrotorsion. And, similarly, an excessive angle of torsion produces a state termed excessive antetorsion. It is pertinent to emphasize that torsional growth is manifested as a twisting of bone resulting in a change of the bone's shape.

There is another growth pattern occurring within the upper segment, e.g., the positional migrations of the femur within the hip joint. At birth we find the femur lying on its side within the acetabulum, the head and neck being angled approximately 60 degrees anteriorly from the frontal plane of the pelvis (Fig. 4). We call this state anteversion, because the head and neck of the femur are

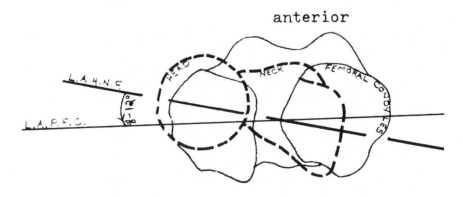

Figure 1.

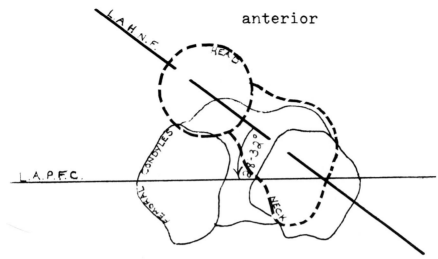

Figure 2.

anteriorly positioned with respect to the frontal plane of the pelvis. It is this relationship that makes the newborn child very susceptible to hip dislocations. For example, hip dysplasias in an alarming number of infants seen at the Ohio Clinic of Podiatric Medicine are subsequently diagnosed as iatrogenically induced. It is not uncommon to find an adducted gait or excessive metatarsus adductus treated with mechanical devices that externally rotate the limb at the hip joint. In young infants, this exogenous rotation can force the head of the femur out of the acetabulum. Indeed, Jacobs (1960) and Colonna (1958) were among the first to note this correlation. Jacobs reported that in examining 300 infants with excessive metatarsus adductus, 10 per cent had concomitant hip dislocations.

This 60 degrees of anteversion present at birth reduces to an adult value of 8-12 degrees (Fig. 5). We commonly refer to this angle as the anterior angle of declination. Any angle less than the normal adult value is termed a posterior angle of declination and the associated state as retroversion. Any angle in excess of the adult value is termed an excessive anterior angle of declination and the resulting condition is called excessive anteversion. During the normal positional migrations within the upper segment, we find the femur internally rotating 48-52 degrees at the hip joint (Fig. 6). This takes place independently of the concurrent torsional growth seen within the shaft of the femur. It must be remembered that anteversion refers to a positional relationship, e.g., a bone-to-bone comparison of the femur to the pelvis within the hip joint. The adult value is usually reached by the time the child has reached his sixth birthday.

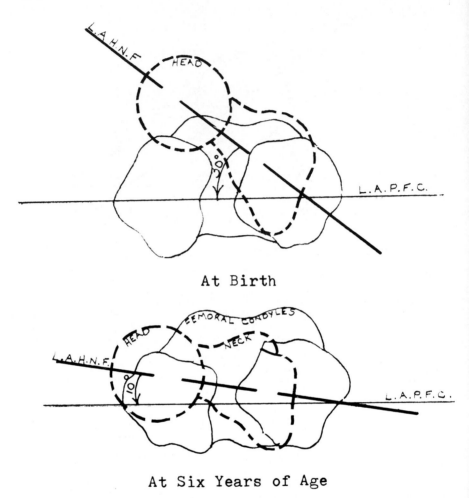

At Birth

At Six Years of Age

Figure 3.

The hip joint's neutral position is defined as that point from which the femur can internally and externally rotate the same number of degrees. Keeping in mind the concomitant events of antetorsion and anteversion, we can easily appreciate why the neutral position of the hip joint at birth places the knee 30 degrees externally rotated on the transverse plane (relative to the frontal plane), while in the adult the hip joint's neutral position places the knee directly on the frontal plane (Fig. 7 and Fig. 8).

Clinically, a pigeon-toed gait is one of the most common findings seen in children. Eighty-five out of 100 times it is due to an excessive amount of

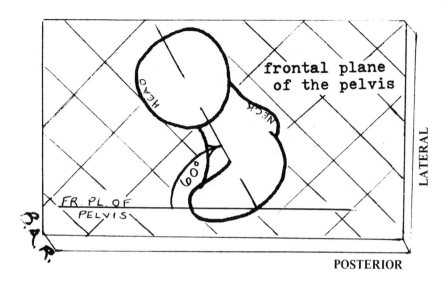

Figure 4.

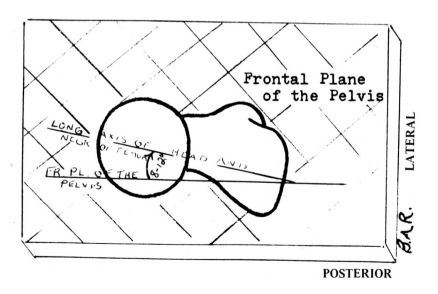

Figure 5.

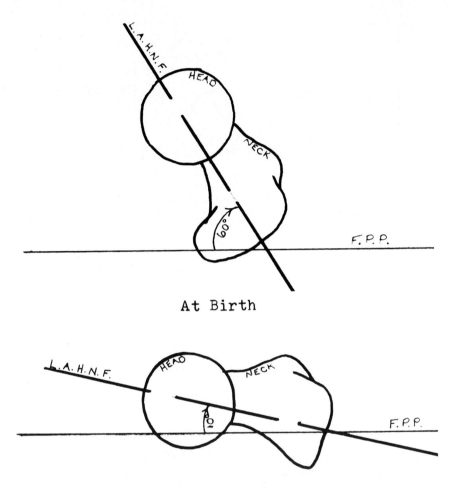

At Birth

Figure 6.

antetorsion (internal femoral torsion) present at birth, e.g., some children start off with an antetorsion greater than the normal 30 degrees (Nicholas, 1934). This means by the time the child first starts to walk, there is still a certain degree of excessive antetorsion left. Occasionally, the bony structure of the femur is normal at birth, but the postnatal torsional growth is stunted. Why this happens, we don't know. However, either condition is manifested clinically as an inwardly rotated gait which the layman identifies as a pigeon-toed child. When we passively rotate the hip joint through its entire range of motion we find that the limbs rotate inwardly and have a restricted outward range of motion with both the hip flexed and extended (Fig. 9). We can determine the amount of

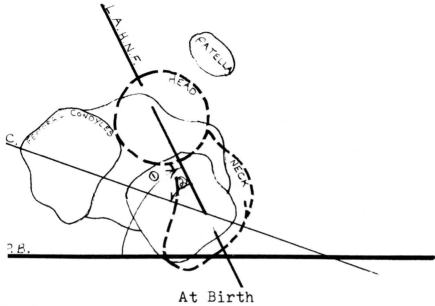

At Birth

Figure 7.

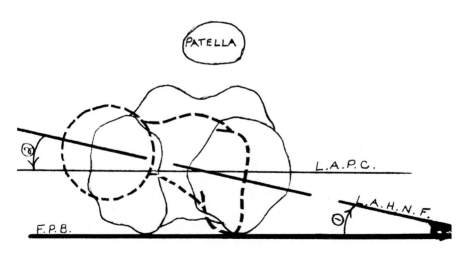

At Six Years of Age

Figure 8.

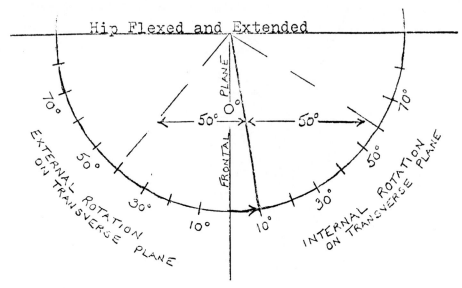

Figure 9.

excessive antetorsion present by placing the hip joint in its neutral position and noting the amount of inward rotation of the posterior condyles of the femur. Normally they should lie directly on the frontal plane (if the child is over the age of six).

Most children will outgrow their excessive antetorsion sooner or later. There are two major growth times for the reduction of this torque: before the age of six and between the ages of 10 to 14. This means if a child of eight is presented to you with an in-toeing gait problem, and through your clinical examination and history you diagnose it as an internal femoral torsion deformity, you can advise the parents that their child will probably outgrow the affliction before he reaches his 15th birthday.

Unfortunately, many of these children are treated by clinicians who do not have a full awareness of the problem. Generally, such cases are treated by a device which substitutes a maximally pronated and subluxed foot for the pigeon-toeing gait. Functional orthotics create motion within the joints; they do not affect torques. By applying a device to the foot, we create motion within the talocalcaneal and midtarsal joints. By applying a device to the leg, we create motion within the hip joint. The easiest way to cause excessive pronation and subluxation of the foot is to place a lateral wedge on the heel of the shoe when the intrinsic structure of the foot is normal. At heel contact the calcaneus is immediately everted which, in turn, unlocks the midtarsal joint enabling the forefoot to maximally pronate upon the rearfoot. The second easiest way to cause foot pronation is to put on a Brachman's skate. This device was originally designed for spastic children, and is excellent for this purpose. However, when applied to a normal child who has an abnormal torque of the femur, as the patient tries to ambulate with his feet forcibly turned outward, his feet maximally pronate. The third easiest way to create closed kinetic chain pronation is to use a Denis-Browne splint. The end result in all of the above therapies is that the child toes in less, but the excessive torque is still there and the child now has a foot whose structural integrity has been destroyed.

To recapitulate, mechanical devices do not effect torques. The only way torques can be changed is by performing a derotatory osteotomy or by simply letting the child outgrow it. Fortunately, it is very rare to find an adult who has sufficient internal femoral torsion to leave him pigeon-toed. Most adults who toe in do so due to a lack of tibial torsion.

Sometimes the parents insist so vehemently that their child be treated that we do so in lieu of them being treated by someone who might inadvertently harm the foot. We treat this affliction palliatively being fully cognizant that in time it will reduce by itself. We direct our treatment toward having the patients function with their hip in an externally rotated position. This will accommodate for the excessive internal femoral torsion without disturbing the structure of the foot. Several mechanical devices are available which create movement within the hip joint without disturbing the bony configuration of the foot. This is accomplished by first supinating the foot which, as demonstrated by Elftman (1960) and Zitzylsperger (1960), locks the foot. With the foot so positioned, an exogenous pronatory force can be safely applied to the limb without destroying the structural integrity of the foot. Ganley's Splint, for example, first supinates the foot maximally and then turns the entire limb outward using the foot as the lever. McGlamry has a device in which he ties the heels together and then forces the knees apart with the knee joint flexed. This forces the patient to turn his femur outward at the hip joint without pronating the foot. Or a torque heel, when walked upon, externally rotates the angle of gait by about 5 degrees at the hip joint. However, it must be replaced every few months.

Another dysplasia we see clinically is an excessive abducted gait due to excessive anteversion, e.g., external femoral position. This is a fairly common clinical entity and is treated by using a device which rotates both the limb and foot inwardly. We do not have to worry about dislocating the foot because by turning the foot medially we are supinating it, and rearfoot supination locks the forefoot. The patient responds miraculously to treatment because the limb is being forced in the same direction that it normally develops. Axiomatically, positional deformities respond to orthopedic treatment, torsional deformities do not. In many instances we clinically establish our definitive diagnosis by noting the index of therapeutic resistance exhibited by the affliction.

Our clinical criterion for diagnosing excessive anteversion is based on three objective findings: (1) the patient displays an excessive abducted gait, (2) the condition proves retractable, and (3) if the positional change is due to a contracture state of a specific muscle, a discrepancy in the transverse plane rotation of the femur is noted with the hip joint flexed and extended (Fig. 10). If the hip joint externally rotates more with the patient sitting up and the knee

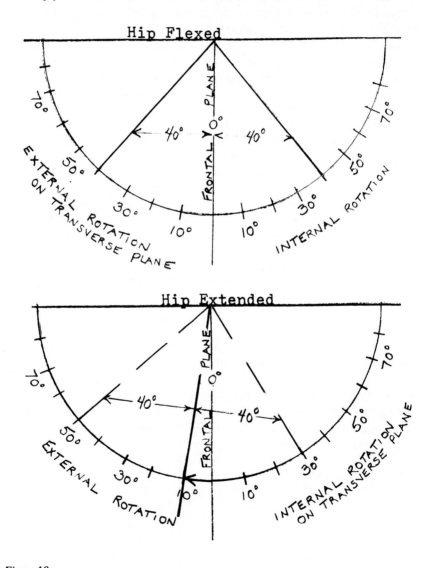

Figure 10.

joint flexed (thus relaxing the hip flexors), we might suspect a contracture of the iliopsoas muscle. On the other hand, if the hip joint externally rotates more with the patient lying down and the knee joint flexed (thus relaxing the hip extensors), we suspect a contracture of the gluteus maximus and minimus. Finally, there may be no muscular involvement. It may be due to either a retention of the juvenile femoral position or an excessive anteversion present at birth, which was simply too much to completely reduce to a normal adult value. Either of the above, if seen in a young adult, can clinically mimic a torsional deformity. In these instances, the differential diagnosis is based solely on the patient's response to therapy.

Some authors (i.e., Giannestras, Kite) have incriminated frog-like sleeping positions as a predisposing factor in excessive out-toeing gait deformities. This author is in complete agreement if one is dealing with a positional anomaly at the hip joint. The frog-like position assumed by some infants during somnolence creates a dynamic imbalance. In this position, the thighs are kept at a right angle to the pelvis and the knees are flexed. Concurrently the limbs are turned outward on the transverse plane (Fig. 11). This places the hip's internal rotators on a stretch while the external rotators are relaxed. Physiologically the muscle that is stretched loses a little power, and the one that is contracted gains a little power. The end result is a muscular imbalance that can delay the normal ontogenetic positional development of the femur, or it can enhance an already prevalent anteversional deformity of the limb.

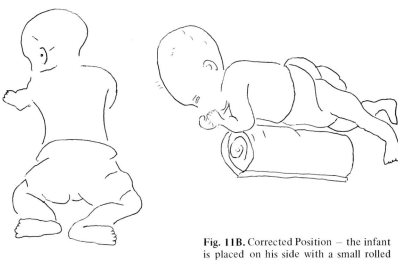

Fig. 11A. Frog-like Position.

Fig. 11B. Corrected Position – the infant is placed on his side with a small rolled towel placed anterior to his abdomen to prevent the child from rolling onto his abdomen.

A third type of dysplasia we see clinically is an in-toeing gait due to
retroversion, e.g., internal femoral position (Fig. 12). We have only seen this
condition in spastic children where either the adductor muscle group or the
medial hamstrings were in a state of clonic spasm. Spastic children must be
handled in an entirely different manner than normal children. What we try to do

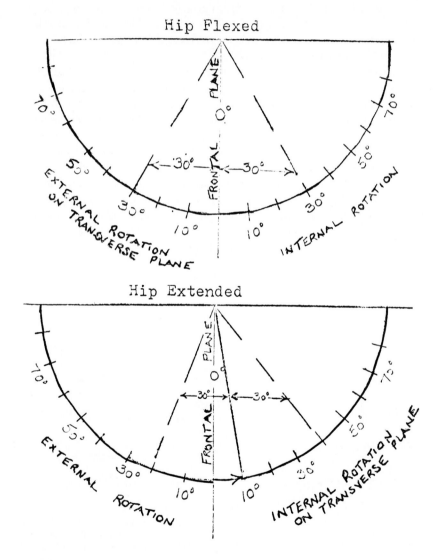

Figure 12.

is to rotate the limb outward at the hip joint by use of a Brachman Skate. Here we are not too concerned about pronating the foot because a spastic child has more problems than just abnormal foot mechanics. In retrospect, this is why when a child is presented to us with a pigeon-toed gait but is normal in other respects, we suspect an antetorsional problem and not a retroversional deformity.

The fourth and last possible type of transverse plane dysplasia which can occur in the upper segment is excessive out-toeing due to retrotorsion, e.g., external femoral torsion (Fig. 13). This clinical identity is rarely seen in children under ten and usually does not manifest itself until after the child has reached puberty. Retrotorsion represents an exaggerated torsional growth within the femur, and being a torsional problem, does not respond to functional devices. For all intents and purposes, this dysplasia is uncorrectable short of surgery. Fortunately, external femoral torsion by itself does not cause severe foot problems. What does occur is at whole foot contact the linear progression of weight falls medially with respect to the longitudinal axis of the foot. As the leg rotates over the foot, it (the leg) rolls around the foot thereby producing a retrograde pronatory force upon the foot. This causes the patient to roll off the medial aspect of the hallux instead of propelling straight off of it. But this is not an active pronatory force. It is a reverse force and, by itself, may produce arch strain and some moderate callus formation, but does not cause any severe symptomatology. The patient displays a strange appearing gait pattern, but is relatively asymptomatic.

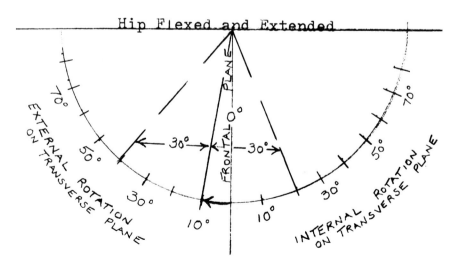

Figure 13.

When examining the transverse plane rotation at the hip joint, the moevement patterns should be bilaterally symmetrical; that is, if the right limb externally and internally rotates 40 degrees, the left limb should also circumscribe an arc of 40 degrees externally and internally. Conversely, a difference in the range of motion of one limb relative to the other – this is not to be confused with an asymmetrical range of motion occurring within the same limb – suggests the presence of a malignant problem: spasm, intra-articular fluid, osteoarthritic proliferative changes, or traumatic changes within the joint. In these instances, a differential diagnosis must be made to isolate the etiological factor and prevent a progression of symptoms.

In summation, antetorsion is internal femoral torsion, anteversion is external femoral position, retrotorsion is external femoral torsion, and retroversion is internal femoral position. The incidence is common, not too common, and rare, in that order. Our treatment is based on three premises: (1) Protect the foot. (2) If the condition is going to outgrow itself, let it. (3) When treating, try to change the position at the hip joint, not within the foot. It is of paramount import that the clinician establish whether he is dealing with a positional or torsional deformity. If torsional (in a child) leave alone, or at most accommodate (i.e., torque heels). If positional, it can be treated and the results are gratifying.

In the lower segment we find the tibia undergoing torsional changes during its normal growth. By looking at the shaft from proximal to distal, comparing the proximal tibial plateau to the distal ankle mortise, we find that at birth the proximal and sital aspects are about parallel with one another; whereas making the same comparison in the adult tibia, we find an angle between the two with the distal aspect being externally deviated about 22-25 degrees (Fig. 14). This angle on the transverse plane is called external tibial torsion. At age one there is about 10 degrees and by age six we consider it to be at its adult value.

Clinically we cannot see nor directly measure tibial torsion, but what we can see clinically is the positional relationship of the fibular malleolus to the tibial malleolus. We define this as malleolar torsion which usually runs concurrently with tibial torsion. Malleolar torsion is measured by bisecting the malleoli distally and comparing this line with the posterior femoral condyles.* The angle formed between these two landmarks gives us a value on malleolar torsion. We consider the adult norm to be between 13-18 degrees.

A crude indication of the presence or lack of malleolar torsion can be ascertained by placing one's thumb and index fingers on the tibial and fibular malleoli, respectively. Normally the thumb should be visibly more anteriorly placed than the index finger. If both digits lie on the frontal plane, we can tentatively diagnose a lack of malleolar torsion.

---

*The tibial plateau cannot be identified topographically hence the posterior femoral condyles are used in its place.

anterior

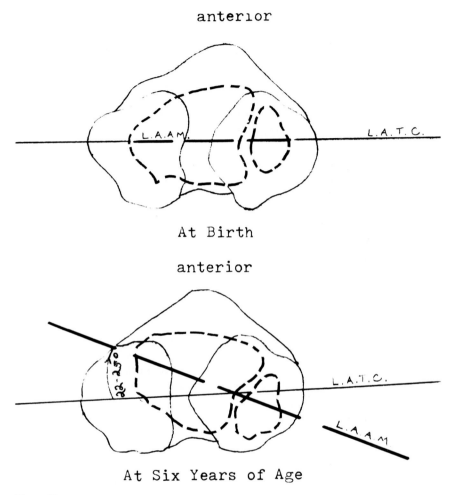

At Birth

anterior

At Six Years of Age

Figure 14.

Any malleolar torsion less than 13-18 degrees is deficient. Any malleolar torsion greater than this normal adult value is considered excessive. We call the latter excessive external malleolar torsion, which can cause an excessive abducted gait. The former is referred to as a lack of malleolar torsion, which can cause a pigeon-toed gait. Excessive external malleolar torsion acts just like external femoral torsion in that (1) you cannot change it, (2) it represents growth too far, and (3) by itself does not produce a severe pronatory force upon the foot. A lack of external malleolar torsion, if severe enough, leaves the individual pigeon-toed. This is the most common cause for an in-toeing gait seen in adults. A pigeon-toed gait can also be caused by internal femoral torsion. We differentiate between these two by observing the spatial positioning of the knee joint while the hip joint is in its neutral position. A lack of external malleolar torsion places the knee joint directly on the frontal plane, whereas excessive antetorsion leaves the knee joint internally rotated on the transverse plane. An adducted gait due to a lack of external malleolar torsion cannot be treated successfully by mechanical devices. At present, the only way we can correct this lack of torsion is by doing a rotatory osteotomy on the shafts of the tibia and fibula. If a mechanical device is used on this type of deformity, we end up with a pronated foot. Once again, with a pigeon-toed child we must differentiate at what level the deformity is located. A diagnosis of saying the child is pigeon-toed is incomplete. We must determine whether the adducted gait pattern is due to antetorsion, lack of external malleolar torsion, or retroversion.

In measuring malleolar torsion we have introduced two other bones, e.g., the fibula and tibia. This sets up a situation where positional changes can occur which are able to simulate a structural deformity. For example, an apparent lack of malleolar torsion can occur from a positional anomaly of the fibula. This means that in some individuals we are unable to measure accurately the torsion present in the lower segment of their limbs. We have two possibilities for failure to be able to match malleolar torsion to true tibial torsion: (1) Some individuals exhibit a hypermobile tibial-fibular relationship, e.g., the proximal amphiarthrodial articulation which is unusually large allows an abnormal amount of mobility. This mobility enables the fibula to move back and forth on the tibia. Measuring malleolar torsion on these individuals is meaningless because the value can be altered by simply changing the position of the fibula with respect to the tibia. (2) In approximately 5% of the patients examined at the Ohio Clinic of Podiatric Medicine, we have found a remarkable transverse plane hypermobility between the tibia and femur at the knee joint with the knee fully extended. This hypermobility allows a condition where the lower segment functions in an inwardly rotated position with respect to the femur at the knee joint. We call this condition a pseudo-lack of malleolar torsion. About 95% of all adducted gait problems seen in adolescents today are due to either a pseudo-lack of malleolar torsion or an excessive antetorsion. Both states can occur concomitantly. One of the worst cases seen at our clinic was in a child who had both.

Since a pseudo-lack of malleolar torsion is a positional deformity, it can be treated successfully by casting. The foot is first placed in a below the knee cast with the foot positioned 90 degrees to the leg. This is allowed to set. The knee is then flexed about 15 degrees, taking extreme care not to introduce a frontal plane deformity with the cast, and the limb is rotated outwardly to its extreme. This position is held while the cast is brought to mid thigh.* This is a two-man

---

*If the cast is not brought up this high, ambulation will loosen the cast, and it will fall off.

casting technique and should not be attempted alone. On the average we've found it necessary to cast for only 4 to 6 weeks to obtain correction. As of June 1970, our success rate has been around 75%. No child has been casted past the age of eight. The casting technique does not eliminate the knee hypermobility. It does direct the lower segment to function in a different position relative to the upper segment. Once this correction is obtained the only post casting treatment required is to prevent the limb from rotating inwardly while the child is asleep. This is accomplished by tieing the back of the heels together.

The foot, or more specifically, the talus, is also undergoing a transverse plane torsional development. At birth an angle of 25-28 degrees is present between the neck and trochlea process of the talus. This torque normally reduces by 3-10 degrees as the child grows older (Fig. 15). Concurrently, there is a transverse plane torsional growth occurring at Lisfranc's articulation. In a neonatal, the metatarsals are medially deviated 20-30 degrees with respect to the lesser tarsal transection. This reduces 5-25 degrees during the normal ontogenetic development of the child (Rothbart, B). A metatarsus adductus between 5-15 degrees is considered normal in an adult.

In a shoe-wearing population, the digits are forced to align to the long axis of the foot. This positional relationship between the phalanges and their corresponding metatarsals is termed digital abductus. Topographically, digital abductus can mask a severe metatarsus adductus pattern.

Possessing the knowledge of the normal transverse plane growth of the limb and foot enables one to understand the rationale behind the statement that a 3 to 7 degree abducted gait in the adult is normal. At birth the sum effect of anteversion and antetorsion within the upper segment places the femoral condyles 28-32 degrees externally deviated on the transverse plane. There is no tibial torsion, and in a shoe-wearing population the metatarsus adductus is clinically sequestered by digital abductus, but the foot deviates 25-28 degrees medially due to the talar torsion. The sum total of these torques places the foot more or less on the sagittal plane when the hip joint is placed in its neutral position.

By the child's sixth birthday, the sum effect of anteversion and antetorsion places the femoral condyles directly on the frontal plane. There is an external tibial torsion of 22-25 degrees, but the foot is deviated 18-22 degrees inwardly from the longitudinal axis of the trochlea due to the talar torsion. The sum effect of this set of torques places the foot 3-7 degrees externally deviated on the transverse plane when the hip joint is placed in its netural position. We see the foot gradually rotated outward as the child matures.

An infant first learning to walk exhibits an excessive abducted gait. The hip joint's neutral position places the feet on the sagittal plane. However, the child of 2 to 3 years of age does not function around his hip joint's neutral position. Due to his poorly developed sense of balance, he must volitionally externally

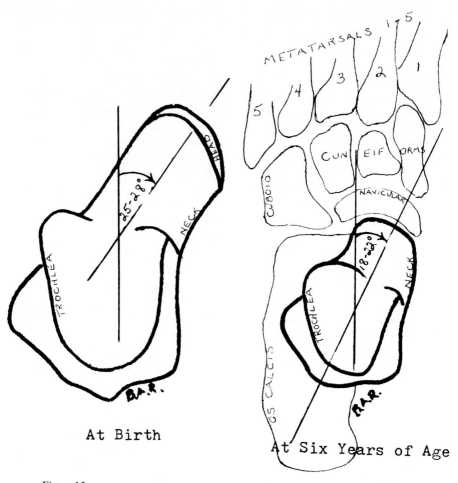

Figure 15.

rotate his feet (hence his entire limb) in order to gain a wide base of support. Otherwise, frequent falls are inevitable. As the infant's sense of equilibrium develops, he is able to function more and more around his hip joint's neutral position. This places his feet only slightly abducted with reference to the midline of the body.

It is hoped that this monograph has brought some light on the rationale behind treatment of the transverse plane dysplasias of the lower limb. Although one can treat, as has been unfortunately demonstrated in the past, adducted and abducted gait problems without understanding the ontogenetic development of the limb, more harm than good can be done to the patient and it is the clinician's primary obligation to his patients to have an accurate understanding of etiology before implementing treatment.

Bibliography

Bardeem, C. R.: Studies in the development of the human skeleton of the posterior limb, *Amer. J. Anat.*, Vol. IV, p. 265, 1905.

Colonna, P. C.: Care of the infant with congenital subluxation of the hip, *JAMA*, *166*:715-720, 1958.

Elftman, H.: The transverse tarsal joint and its control, *Clin. Orthop.*, *16*:41-46, 1960.

Elftman, H.; and Manter, J. T.: Evolution of the human foot, *J. Anat.*, *70*, pp. 56-67, 1935.

Giannestras, N. J.: *Foot Disorders*, Philadelphia: Lea and Febiger, 1967.

Jacobs, J. E.: Metatarsus varus and hip dysplasia, *Clin. Orthop.*, *16*:203-213, 1960.

Kite, J. H.: Torsion of the lower extremities in small children, *J. Bone, J. Surg.*, *36-A*:511-520, 1954.

Kite, H. H.: Flat feet and lateral rotation of legs in young children, *J. Internat. Coll. Surg.*, *25*:77-84, 1956.

Nachlas, I. W.: Medial Torsion of the leg, *Arch. Surg.*, *28:*909-919, 1934.

Rothbart, B.: *Biomechanics of the Lower Limb*, unpublished manuscript.

Schultz, A. H.: Foetal growth of man, *Amer. J. Phys. Anthrop.*, Vol. 6, 1923.

Topical Control of Infection on Gangrenous Lesions of the Extremities

Stanley Levine

Gangrene of the extremities, and other chronic lesions, can result from arterial insufficiency, local trauma, infection, vascular stasis, occlusion, or release of toxic bacterial products.[1,2] Because of their specific vascular pathology, diabetics are especially prone to the development of any of the above conditions, and hence to gangrenous and other lesions of the extremities.[3] Conservative treatment of the gangrene, combined with systemic antibiotics to prevent or treat local infecions, is often difficult, particularly in the presence of diabetic microangiopathy.[4]

Local infection presents a dual problem in that: 1) the infective organism may be resistant to commonly used antibiotics, and 2) the presence of vascular impairment reduces absorption and distribution of systemic antibiotics to extremities, even when organisms are sensitive to the antibiotic.[5] Topical control of the infection with bandages soaked in an antibacterial solution lethal to organisms commonly implicated in these lesions would appear to be the optimal method for resolving this dual problem. Our experience with povidone-iodine indicates that it is effective for this purpose.

Povidone-iodine is a broad spectrum antiseptic with prolonged microbicidal activity, which produces no appreciable pain even on denuded surfaces.[6] It has proved to be lethal to bacterial strains known to be resistant to antibiotics, and bandages soaked in povidone-iodine solution may be covered with gauze or adhesive bandage to form an occlusive dressing. The present paper reports three cases in which povidone-iodine, in solution* and ointment* form, was effective in controlling longstanding infections in which the offending organisms were resistant to several commonly employed antibiotics.

Stanley Levine, D.P.M., A.A.C.F.S., *Massapequa, New York.*

*Betadine Solution, and Betadine Ointment, each containing 10% povidone-iodine (1% available iodine), provided by The Purdue Frederick Company, Yonkers, N.Y.

Case Reports

Three patients, at the time of referral, had gangrenous lesions on extremities that were uncontrolled and spreading. Similar significant findings were made in all three: 1) a heavy, uncontrolled infection; 2) peripheral vascular disease, and 3) bacteria resistant to commonly-used antibiotics. In vitro studies indicated that povidone-iodine was lethal to the organisms isolated (Table 1).

Case 1: A 73-year old diabetic female with vascular insufficiency of the lower extremities was initially seen on November 18, 1969. Gangrenous lesions on the left foot extended from the first metatarsal head to the fifth metatarsal area. She had been hospitalized in June with gangrene of the left third toe, and the toe and a portion of the metatarsal head had been excised. The wound had not healed and the gangrene had spread on the plantar surface. Infection was heavy. Cultures showed a mixture of *Aerobacter aerogenes, Pseudomonas aeruginosa* and *Proteus mirabilis,* which demonstrated resistance to: cephaloridine, ampicillin, chloromycetin, colistin, kanamycin, oxytetracycline, polymyxin B, streptomycin, tetracycline and vibromycin.

Occlusive wet dressings soaked in povidone-iodine solution were applied continuously, bringing the infection under control in two weeks. Necrotic tissue was debrided and the povidone-iodine wet dressings maintained for another five weeks. On December 30 the patient became ambulatory and the wet dressings were replaced by povidone-iodine ointment, with bandages changed twice daily. Discharged January 16, 1970, the patient was seen regularly through June. There was no further evidence of gangrene.

Case 2: A 76-year old female with vascular insufficiency and gangrenous lesions extending from the left fifth toe to the hallux and second toe was seen initially on September 25, 1970. The gangrene had developed in the fifth toe a

TABLE 1. *In vitro* Killing Time of PVP-I Against
Types of Organisms Implicated in Three Cases

Patient	Bacteria Isolated	Killing Time[14,15] (vs. Same Organisms)	
		PVP-I Solution	PVP-I Ointment
#1	(Mixed infection)		
	Aerobacter aerogenes	15 Sec.	30 sec.
	Pseudomonas aeruginosa	15 - 30 sec.	60 sec.
	Proteus mirabilis	30 sec.	30 sec.
#2	*Staphylococus aureus* (coagulase positive)	15 - 30 sec.	60 sec.
#3	*Pseudomonas aeruginosa*	15 - 30 sec.	60 sec.

year earlier following severe trauma. Sympathectomy and amputation of the toe at the metatarsal joint had failed to prevent spread of the gangrene. The fifth metatarsal head protruded through an oozing wound, and some plantar tissue had become necrotized. Culture indicated *Staphylococcus aureus* (coagulase positive), resistant to: erythromycin, ampicillin, chloromycetin, colistin, gentamicin, kanamycin, lincomycin, methicillin, oxacillin and demeclocycline.

Debridement of necrotic tissue was followed by an occlusive wet dressing soaked with povidone-iodine solution. Infection was controlled in two weeks and vasodilators administered. Debridement and the wet dressings were continued, the fifth metatarsal head excised, the wound closed and the second toe amputated. Gangrenous tissue on the hallux was excised. Povidone-iodine ointment dressings replaced the wet dressing when the patient became ambulatory. Two months later plantar lesions were healed, gangrene and infection were controlled, and skin color was approaching normal.

Case 3: A 46-year old diabetic female presented with gangrenous lesions on left heel, hallux, distal plantar aspect and medial side of second toe. An infection on the heel had spread. There was a circular black area 4 cm in diameter, surface tissue was dead and partially mummified, and areas of necrotic fat tissue lay underneath. Culture revealed *Pseudomonas aeruginosa,* resistant to several antibiotics, but sensitive to: chlortetracycline, oxytetracycline and doxycycline.

Wound debridement was followed by application of wet dressings soaked with povidone-iodine solution. Vasodilators were administered, and a high protein diet supplemented with high potency vitamins prescribed. Ambulation was restricted. After 15 days of continuous wet dressings, povidone-iodine ointment dressings were substituted. Evidence of gangrene has subsided and improvement has been steady.

Summary and Conclusion

Gangrenous lesions of the extremities are often complicated by invasion of infective organisms, especially so in diabetic individuals or people with peripheral vascular disease. Further complications include resistance of these organisms to commonly employed antibiotics. In cases where the infective agent is sensitive to systemic antibiotics, vascular impairment may prevent adequate distribution to affected extremities. Treatment requires elimination of the infection and debridement of necrotic tissue. Use of povidone-iodine ointment, employed sequentially, is an effective means of controlling infection on gangrenous lesions.

References

1. Rahat, J. J., Jr., et al.: Thrombocytopenia and symmetrical peripheral gangrene associated with Staphylococcal and Streptococcal Bacteremia. *Ann. Intern. Med.* 39:35-43 (July), 1968.

2. Rosenberg, N.: Long term antibiotic administration for localized gangrene. *Amer. Surg.* *35*:348-350 (May), 1969.

3. Rhodes, E. L.: Dermatological problems in the diabetic patient. *Geriatrics 23*:132-136 (July), 1968.

4. Lopez, J. E., et al.: Local insulin for diabetic gangrene. *Lancet 1*:1199 (June), 1968.

5. Robertson, P. D.: Foot lesions in diabetics. *Med. Times 96*:592-597 (June), 1968.

6. McKnight, A. G.: A clinical trial of povidone-iodine in the treatment of chronic leg ulcers. *Practitioners 195*:230-234 (Aug.), 1965.

7. VanderWyk, R. W.: Killing efficiency of an iodophor. Scientific Exhibit presented to Aerospace Medical Association Meeting, Wash., D.C., April 10-13, 1967.

8. Personal communication from the Medical Department, The Purdue Frederick Company, Yonkers, N.Y.

A Clinical Study of the Phalangeal Stance Reflex

Stanley V. Michota and Franklin A. Michota

This quantitative study examines the plantar surface of the foot during the standing position, as it reflects the stress of body weight and the force of equilibrium which are superimposed upon it.

The examination of the plantar surface of the foot is not new. Inked footprints of newborn infants have received a widespread acceptance as a means of identification. Also, some foot impressions of newborn infants have elicited the presence of congenital abnormalities, such as, bilateral or unilateral talipes equinovarus, metatarsus varus or primus.

In a recent report found in the *Journal of Bone and Joint Surgery*, Dr. L. M. Japas of Argentina, discusses "Photopodograms," (weightbearing footprints), which he used pre and postoperatively in the surgical management of a pes cavus type foot. The use of a wet-sole footprint for a pes cavus weightbearing examination admittedly had its drawbacks.

In a recent translation of a book entitled, *Walking and Limping*, authored by Drs. R. J. and P. Ducroquet, orthopedic surgeons of France, we find a description of a "glass cage," and how it was used for examinations of normal and abnormal movements of arms, lower extremities, trunk and head of subjects during locomotion. The "glass cage" made use of reflecting mirrors placed in strategic locations, which enabled the examiners to observe upright subjects from all angles.

The "glass cage" principle has been applied in this study of the plantar surface of 272 subjects, examined while standing in an upright position. A visual examination of the sole of the weightbearing foot, during the upright standing position, can provide the examiner with valuable information of aberrations of structural, functional, and prehensile competency of the foot, functioning as an integral part of a neuromuscular system in the maintenance of upright equilibirum.

During the examination, the subjects stood upon a square cabinet, with a clear, plexiglass top and tilted mirror below it, which reflected the plantar

Stanley V. Michota, D.P.M., *and* Franklin A. Michota, D.P.M., *Toledo, Ohio*

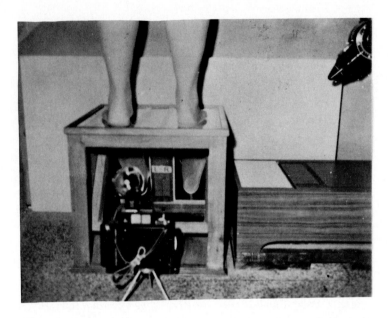

Figure 1.

surface of both feet. The reflected foot prints were then photographed with a Polaroid camera, having a portrait lens, flash attachment and color film.

In studying the role a foot plays during the upright standing position, many authors, among them Basmajian, Brunstrom, Caillet, Mann and Inman, all concur that very few muscles, if any, are innervated. There are contradictory opinions as to muscle activity during upright standing. Some studies have revealed that calorie consumption is present, although minimal, during all upright standing, and that calorie consumption becomes higher during the erect and prolonged standing positions.

Brunstrom, in his book titled *Clinical Kinesiology,* maintains that during the standing position, the metatarsal joints are considered to be the anterior limit of support, while Mann and Inman, in an article titled "Phasic Activity of Intrinsic Muscles of the Foot," state that "during quiet, upright standing, *no* phalangeal activity should be encountered."

However, in this clinical study we find many photographs of footprints of standing subjects, which do reflect phalangeal activity. Therefore, we must conclude that some conditions do prevail which influence kinetic action, with the resultant plantar flexion of the toes.

Subjects examined ranged from 2 through 82 years of age, males and females. Following a study of the photographs of their footprints, it became apparent that congenital, as well as acquired factors involving the foot and leg, do influence the attitude the foot assumes during the upright standing position. Clinical findings confirm the hypothesis that where an anatomical compensation for assisting postural stability and equilibrium was in demand, an automatic plantar flexion of the toes became evident. Thus, during the upright standing position, the plantar toe flexion is now presumed to be the visible kinetic response of a phalangeal stance reflex, whose clinical significance has not been previously reported.

In DeJong's text titled *Neurologic Examination*, we find an illustration of 19 foot and leg stimuli which elicit plantar toe flexion, but none during the upright standing position when a foot is exposed to postural or gravitational demands.

According to Brunstrom, "the degree of stability, during upright standing, depends upon three factors: one, the size of the surface of support; two, the height of the center of gravity above the supporting surface; and three, the location of the center-of-gravity line with respect to the surface of support." He further states that, "the larger the supporting surface and the lower the center of gravity, the greater the stability; the closer the center-of-gravity line falls to the center of the base of support, the better the stability."

We must admit, that in man, the size of the surface of support is relatively small. The question arises, is it possible for the size of the surface of support to be abnormally small? Yes, it is possible. Of the photographs taken of foot impressions of standing subjects, 208 out of 544 revealed footprints with no visible, lateral midtarsal weightbearing area. This diminished or lack of midtarsal compression is a common occurrence in a hollow or pes cavus type foot or a foot which is abnormally pronated. Since the degree of stability depends upon the size of the base of support, obviously, in a pes cavus type or maximally pronated type foot, the optimum condition for maintenance of upright stability does not exist.

We found plantar toe flexion in 193 of the 208 photographs of pes cavus or diminished foot prints. Why was the plantar toe flexion elicited? Because the size of the base of support was abnormally small. Therefore, the automatic neuromuscular system elicited compensatory toe pressure, which increased the size of the base of support. In addition, and possibly of more significance, the phalangeal activity increased a diminished area of sensory perception.

Often overlooked is the contribution the human foot makes, as a prehensile, sensory organ within a complex neuromuscular system. Within the skin of the plantar surface of the foot are found tactile receptors, which contribute significantly to our terrestial awareness. Even with one's eyes closed, one is conscious of one's environment, whether one stands upon an incline, sandy beach or rocky terrain. In other words, an acuity of sensory perception is evident when our feet are in touch with the ground. Since the rate of discharge of afferent nerve impulses from the skin is directly proportionate to the area of

TABLE 1. Incidence of Toe Pressure During Upright Standing

Degree of Compressed Areas	Number Total	Great & Lesser Toes	Great Toe Only	Lesser Toes Only	No Toe Pressure	More Left	More Right
No Lateral Area	208	183	5	5	15		
Asymmetrical Area	200	154	11	17	18	118	82
Wide Area	104	60	10	10	24		
Slight Lateral Area	32	28			4		
TOTAL	544	410	15	15	48		

the surface of the skin which is compressed or in touch with the environment, the compensatory plantar-flexion of the toes adds immeasureably to a diminished sensory base of support.

As an example, a 62-year-old male was examined, with a 24-year history of diabetes, occupation furrier, having a foot problem with ischemia, several

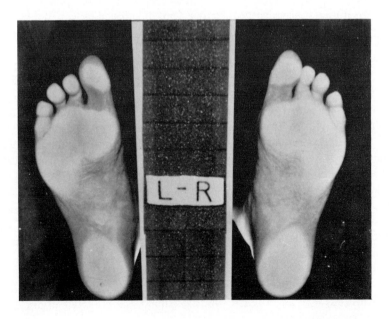

Figure 2.

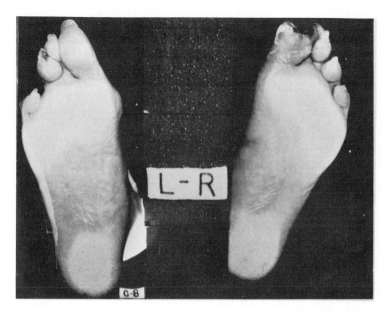

Figure 3.

gangrenous toes, and experiencing very little pain. Photographs of his foot prints revealed a bilateral, diminished weightbearing area, demonstrating that an optimum base of support for postural stability did not exist. In the photographs of his foot prints we found compensatory phalangeal involvement. We must admit that the diabetic condition, with its early angiopathy and advanced neuropathy, were factors which predisposed to the gangrenous toes. Knowing what we know now, about compensatory phalangeal activity, this individual throughout the years, had two other factors which adversely affected his degree of stability and innervated excessive toe motion. First, the size of support was diminished, with an associated diminished area of sensory perception. Secondly, the individual's occupation as a furrier necessitated working with his hands in front of his body, an occupational postural position which moved the center of gravity line anteriorly, and also innervated plantarflexion of the toes. The prolonged contraction of muscles during the standing position, associated with the additional toe activity for the maintenance of equilibrium, created a demand for circulation, which, in this instance, was greater than the supply.

The need for sensory perception and a large base of support is graphically demonstrated in the upright posture of a toddler. Most photographs of toddlers' footprints where the neuromuscular system is not fully coordinated or intact, show a large base of support, a pseudo-pes-planus weightbearing surface, with

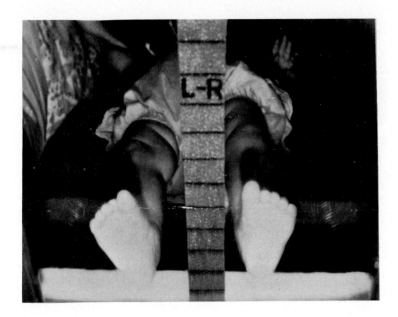

Figure 4.

all, or most all of the toes plantarflexed. Since bipedal upright standing is apparently a learned accomplishment, the need for a large base of support as well as a need for a large area of sensory, prehensile perception, is the endowment of most children, during their impressionable, developing years. In addition, during a toddler's upright position, its outstretched arms and wide stance favorably influence postural stability and equilibrium.

It is obvious that the upright standing position of a biped human does not offer a great deal of stability because the surface of support is relatively small, and the center of gravity of the body lies relatively high, about the level of S 1 and S 2. However, with respect to the third criteria mentioned for maintenance of upright equilibrium, some optimum conditions do exist. The body possesses an automatic neuromuscular mechanism, which maintains the center of gravity line close to the center of the base of support. The question arises, is it possible during the standing position, for the center of gravity line to shift away from the center of the base of support to be reflected as an abnormality? Yes, it is possible.

In 200 photographs we found the presence of asymmetrical footprints, where a larger area of compression was visible, either in the left or right footprint of the standing subject. The asymmetrical footprints frequently were characteristic of unequal leg lengths. A high percentage (182 of 200)

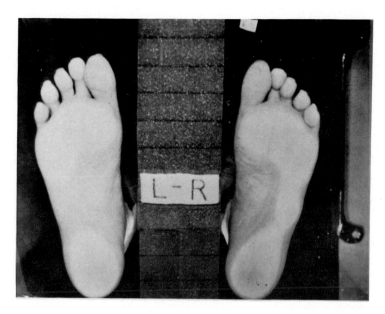

Figure 5.

asymmetrical footprints demonstrated phalangeal activity. Also, the shorter limb demonstrated a larger area of compression, and significantly, greater phalangeal involvement.

It was found that some photographs of footprints of seemingly adequate size and equal weightbearing surface also revealed plantar toe flexion. In the majority of these subjects, although the weightbearing surface was not diminished or asymmetrical, subsequent examination revealed the foot to be functionally or structurally unstable.

Since the phalangeal stance reflex when elicited was found to be more prevalent in photographs of diminished or asymmetrical footprints, subjects who did not demonstrate some phalangeal activity under these conditions frequently demonstrated inhibitory factors which curtailed the compensatory toe function. Examination of these subjects often elicited functional or structural anomalies such as extensive phalangeal contractures and ankylosis. The subjects with diminished or asymmetrical footprints that were unable to elicit phalangeal activity compensated their postural demands at a higher level of the body. Frequently, these individuals complained of knee pain, leg cramps, fatigue and back discomfort.

Physiologically speaking, the presence of phalangeal involvement during the upright standing position is deemed highly significant. The kinetic response answering gravitational demands, indicated that the subject was no longer standing in a completely relaxed manner, that a physical response for assisting postural stability was being reflected by muscle activity and energy expenditure.

The question arises, is it possible to diminish the phalangeal activity by modifying some factors which adversely effect postural stability? Yes, it is possible. Photographs of the plantar surface of individuals while standing upon clear, contour, acrylic inlays demonstrated that the diminished weightbearing area can be increased, the stability improved, and phalangeal activity lessened, provided dorsal flexion of the ankle is not restricted. A study of stability at the Myo-Dynamic Laboratory at the Rochester School of Medicine reported that any shoe which is not as flat as the floor, will improve the stability of a pes cavus type foot. However, although the size or area of support is increased, an individual wearing high heels consumes more oxygen, as the center of gravity shifts anteriorly and innervates the plantar flexors.

Phalangeal activity was curtailed significantly in standing subjects when a forefoot varus attitude was accommodated by applying biomechanic principles. The accommodation of a short leg syndrome improved stability and phalangeal activity was diminished in some subjects.

Photographs have shown that clasping the hands in front of the body during the standing position will innervate plantar flexion of the toes. This type of occupational attitude, with the hands in front of the body during upright standing, predisposes toward forefoot pathology. Conversely, when the hands

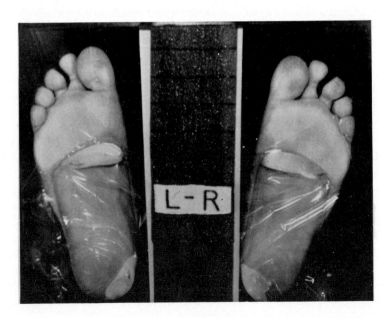

Figure 6.

are clasped behind the body during upright standing, phalangeal activity is diminished. It is not surprising that "Parade Rest" is a welcome command from a position of "Attention" to a member of the Armed Forces. The wide stance, as well as clasping the hands behind the body, is a postural attitude "of quiet upright standing, where *no* phalangeal activity should be encountered."

In summary, it is apparent that plantar toe flexion is innervated by a predictable phalangeal stance reflex, part of an automatic neuromuscular mechanism, where there are significant aberrations in factors which determine the degree of postural stability and equilibrium. The early detection and management of controllable factors which adversely affect postural stability can result in a more efficient base of support, one which performs its function with minimal energy expenditure, while satisfying the gravitational, sensory and postural demands of a biped human, standing in space in an upright position.

References

1 Basmajian, J. V., and Stecko, G.: Role of Muscles in Arch Support of Foot (An Electromyographic Study). *J. Bone and Joint Surg.*, Vol. 45A – No. 6 Sept. 1963.
2 Brunstromm, S.: *Clinical Kinesiology*, F. A. Davis Company, 1966: 219-273.
3 Caillet, R.: Foot and Ankle Pain, F. A. Davis Co., 1968, pp. 18-20, 45.
4 DeJong, R. N.: *The Neurologic Examination*, New York: Hoeber-Harper, 1958, p. 594.
5 Ducroquet, R. J., and Ducroquet, P.: *Walking and Limping*, (Trans. Hunter, S., and Hunter, J.). J. P. Lippincott Co., 1965, pp. 8-20.
6 Elftman, H.: Biomechanics of Muscle, *J. Bone and Joint Surg.*, Vol. 46A, 2:363, 1966.
7 Inman, V. T.: Human Locomotion, *Canad. Med. Ass. J.*, May, 1966, Vol. 94.
8 Japas, L. M.: Surgical Treatment of Pes Cavus (Photopodograms Pre & Post Op), *J. Bone and Joint Surg.*, Vol. 50A-15, July, 1968.
9 Mann, R., and Inman, V. T.: Phasic Activity of Intrinsic Muscles of the Foot, *J. Bone and Joint Surg.*, Vol. 46A, 3:469-481, 1964.
10 McCauley, J., Jr., Luskin, R., and Bromley, J.: Recurrence in Congenital Metatarsus Varus, *J. Bone and Joint Surg.* Vol. 46A, 3:525, 1964.
11 Mathews, D. K., and Wooten, E. P.: *Arch. Physiol. Med. and Rehabilit.* Vol. 44, Oct. 1963.
12 Michota, S. V.: Weight-bearing Error Diagnosed and Recorded by Color Photography, *Podiatry News*, Vol. 5, No. 5, 1967.
13 Pepin, W. A., and Marchand, E. R.: Mechanics of Weight Bearing, (Report), *Podiatry News* Vol. 8, No. 2.
14 Schartz, R. P., Heath, A. L., Morgan, D. W., and Towns, R. C.: Analysis of Recorded Variables of Walking Patterns, *J. Bone and Joint Surg.* Vol. 46A: 333, March, 1964.
15 Sgarlato, T. E.: Function of the Foot and its Effect Upon Posture, Continuing Education Seminar, 1969 Program Notes.
16 Sutherland, D. H.: An Electromyographic Study of the Plantar Flexors of the Ankle, *J. Bone and Joint Surg.* Vol. 48A: 67, 1967.
17 Wechsler, I. S.: *Clinical Neurology, Reflexes*. W. B. Saunders, 1958, pp. 16-24.

Axial Rotation of the First Metatarsal as a Factor in Hallux Valgus

Richard A. Maldin

Introduction

More than a hundred years ago, Volkman (1856) complained that the "affection" that "not only deforms the foot in a most clumsy way but also makes the gait uncertain and continuous walking painful," had not been receiving the attention it deserved.[1] Since then, what we now refer to as hallux valgus has received a great deal of attention but little elucidation as to definitive etiology or to possible preventive medicine.

Boneface, in 1895, grouped the divergent concepts under four classes: mechanical, muscular, diathesque and anatomical. Walsam and Hughes, in the same year, spoke of ligamentous and arthritic causes, while Mouchet in 1922 discussed hereditary and trophic disturbances as etiologic factors in hallux valgus.[2] More recently, several orthopedic researchers have beeen referring to an axial rotation of the first metatarsal as both a factor and a finding in cases of hallux valgus formation.

This study was conducted to determine and to measure this so-called "axial rotation" of the first metatarsal as found in patients suffering from varying degrees of hallux valgus and to compare this to a "normal" but younger group of subjects. Using a new positioning device and a new radiographic technique to demonstrate the plantar aspect of the forefoot in static stance, it was hoped to correlate axial rotation of the first metatarsal with measurements taken from dorsal-plantar radiographs.[3]

Methods and Materials

Using the simple positioning device as described by Downey and Dorothy in their article in the April, 1969 issue of the *Journal of the American Podiatry*

Richard A. Maldin, D.P.M. *Bridgeport, Connecticut.*

Association, it was possible to produce a radiographic film demonstrating the relationship of the plantar metatarsal heads to the transverse plane in the base and the angle of gait during stance. This positioning device, shown in Figure 1 consists of a hardwood base measuring 4-1/2″ × 14″ × 1″; a balsa wood sliding heel wedge angled 12° and measuring 4-5/8″ × 6″; and a toe lift consisting of a wedge 1-1/2″ × 1 ″ with an angle of approximately 32°.[4] An intensifying cassette was used, as shown in the diagrams on the following pages, for the axial radiographs; for the dorsal-plantar pictures a leatherette film holder was simply positioned on the floor for the patient to stand upon.

For both the axial and the dorsal-plantar radiographs, 10″ × 12″ Kodak RP/A X-Omat Medical X-Ray film with tinted estar and a safety base was used (Fig. 2).

Patient Position

"The patient stands for the axial view with the left foot placed perpendicular to the film and the toes touching the film. The right foot is on the device placed in the base of gait but not exposed at this time. The toes are raised on the anterior wedge allowing the metatarsals to rest on the base. The heel wedge is brought forward to raise the plantar soft tissue and the heel above the metatarsal

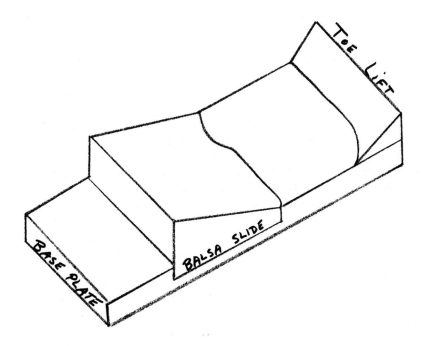

Figure 1. Positioning device.

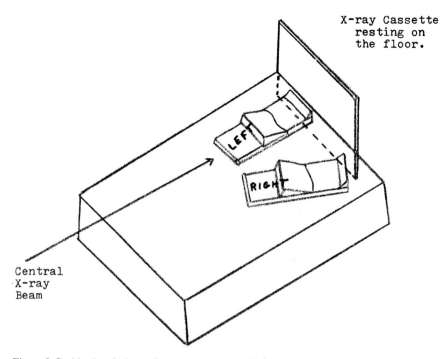

**X-ray Cassette
resting on
the floor.**

**Central
X-ray
Beam**

Figure 2. Positioning device and cassette as arranged for exposure.

heads to reduce superimposition and to assume a more natural stance position (Fig. 3). The patient stands with equal weight on both feet during the exposure as shown in the photographs. The procedure was then repeated for the radiograph of the right foot."[5]

The angle of the central ray was of critical importance for both the axial and the dorsal-plantar views (Fig. 4). For the axial radiograph, the central ray was set at 90° to the film and centered on the midline of the posterior aspect of the foot. In the dorsal-plantar exposure, the central ray was angled at 15° and centered on the base of the third metatarsal (Fig. 5).

Exposure and Developing

For both radiographs a Norelco 50 Kilovolt x-ray machine was used. The film-tube distance used was twenty inches with an exposure time of two and a half seconds for both angles. The developing time was five minutes at 68° temperature with normal solutions.

Measurements

An objective measure of the valgus deformity on the plantar radiograph was the first requisite in defining the terms of reference of this paper. Four distinct

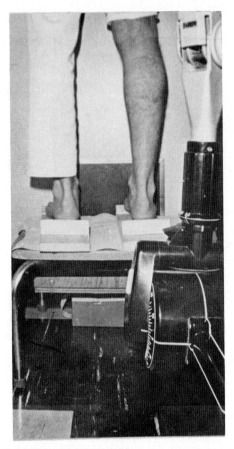

Figure 3. Posterior view of the axial positioning.

measurements were taken from the dorsal-plantar x-rays as diagrammed in Figure 6. These consisted of:

1. *Angle of Metatarsus Adductus.* This is the angle formed by the line bisecting the shaft of the second metatarsal with the line that is perpendicular to the bisection of the lesser tarsus.

2. *Angle of Hallux Valgus.* This is the angle formed by the lines bisecting the first metatarsal and the line bisecting the proximal phalange.

3. *Angle Between the First Metatarsal and the Lesser Tarsus Perpendicular.* This is the angle formed by the line bisecting the first metatarsal with the line perpendicular to the lesser tarsus bisection.

4. *Angle Between the First and Second Metatarsals.* This is the angle formed by the lines bisecting the shafts of the first and second metatarsals respectively.

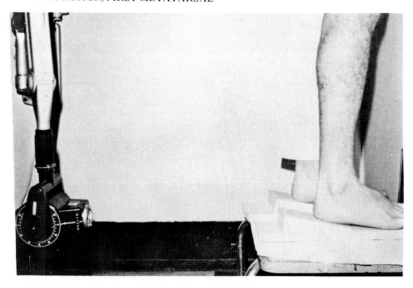

Figure 4. Lateral view of the axial positioning.

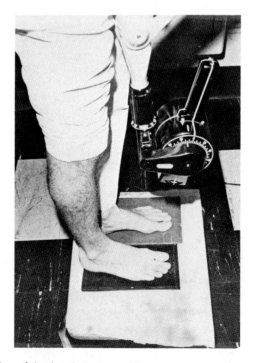

Figure 5. Lateral view of the dorsal-plantar positioning.

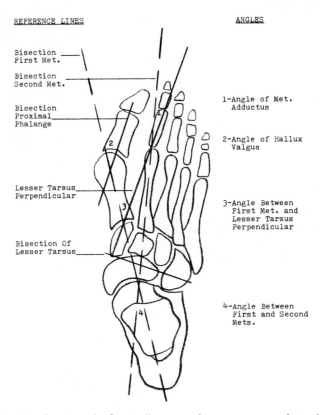

Figure 6. Schematic of angles and reference lines as used to measure x-ray determination.

Having established objective measurements for the dorsal-plantar radiographs, it was next necessary to define the terms of reference as seen on the axial radiographs. Two criteria were decided upon:

1. *Axial Rotation of the First Metatarsal.* Since it was not found possible to make an objective measure of this observation, rotation was therefore simply said to be present or absent.

2. *Displacement of the Sesamoids.* The position of the sesamoids in relation to the head of the first metatarsal was measured by relating the position of the medial sesamoid to the intersesamoid ridge. Five degrees of position were recorded as shown in the series of diagrams in (Fig. 7). Thus, in the first degree sesamoid position, the medial sesamoid is completely on the medial side of the intersesamoid ridge, and this represents the normal position (Fig. 8). On the other hand, in the fifth degree position the medial sesamoid is completely on the lateral side of the ridge, and this represents the extreme of deviation. Degrees two and four represent the medial sesamoid just slightly underlying the

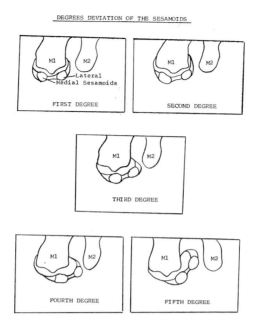

Figure 7. Degrees deviation of the sesamoid.

intersesamoid ridge, while the third degree displacement shows the medial sesamoid to lie directly beneath the intersesamoid ridge (Figs. 9-11).

Discussion

For the purposes of this study, each foot was treated as a unit so that recorded data on the following pages refer to feet and not to subjects unless otherwise stated. Data was recorded from the radiographs of fifty-seven feet. Of these, forty-six were patients with varying degrees of objectively visible hallux valgus; the other eleven cases were of a younger group of patients with no visible signs of hallux valgus and whom it was hoped would approximate a normal for this study.

Before reviewing the recorded data, it must be stated at the outset that the original topic which was entitled: "Axial Rotation of the First Metatarsal in Hallux Valgus" was unsubstantiated by this study. After careful evaluation of all x-rays, it was concluded that no axial rotation of the first metatarsal could be inferred from any of the radiographs. However, the films did clearly reveal a lateral displacement of the sesamoids in the hallux valgus group as well as several other significant points which will be dealt with later.

TABLE 1. Objectively Visible Hallux Valgus Patients

Subject	Angle bt. First & Mets.	Angle of Hallux Valgus	Angle of Met. Adductus	Angle bt. Met-Lesser Tarsus	Degrees Sesamoid Deviation
RS	10	20	11	21	---
	12	23	13	25	---
AW	10	20	14	23	III
	11	24	15	21	III
JG	12	25	16	29	I
	11	21	16	28	II
EC	10	22	13	21	III
	11	25	131	23	IV
CR	11	32	19	22	IV
	11	29	19	20	III
DC	13	53	13	25	V
	—	---	---	---	---
LT	15	30	13	17	III
	13	31	12	25	III
CM	11	29	18	28	IV
AJ	15	17	11	22	II
	7	14	13	17	I
ZT	11	21	8	21	III
	14	30	8	22	IV
JC	15	19	26	40	III
	17	24	17	34	IV
LH	17	11	17	30	II
	13	33	20	28	IV
AW	10	19	14	18	II
	11	28	15	25	IV
ED	14	13	8	14	I
	12	17	8	15	II
LB	13	26	30	36	III
	13	28	28	38	III
FR	10	10	15	27	II
	11	15	25	32	II
CL	12	21	15	18	III
	11	22	12	21	II
EG	16	33	25	32	III
	15	33	32	30	III
EJ	15	26	10	29	IV
	14	19	10	26	III
MM	15	30	15	31	IV
	18	32	17	30	IV
DC	17	40	18	32	V
	19	41	16	36	V

Table 1 – (Continued)

Patients With No Objective Signs of Hallux Valgus

Subject	Angle bt. First & Second Mets.	Angle of Hallux Valgus	Angle of Met. Adductus	Angle bt. Met-Lesser Tarsus Perpend.	Degrees Sesamoid Deviation
MF	12	16	18	28	I
	12	10	15	26	I
MG	9	10	19	24	I
	8	14	15	21	II
WS	11	12	15	20	I
	8	7	20	23	I
JF	12	2	19	28	I
	10	3	12	21	II
AK	10	10	15	25	II
	10	7	15	25	II
LS	11	10	17	26	II
	10	8	16	25	I
MP	9	3	11	20	I
	9	11	12	25	I
MS	10	8	14	24	I
	11	8	15	22	I
AR	11	1	11	17	I

Tabulation of Results

		Patients Exhibiting Hallux Valgus	Patients Not Exhibiting Hallux Valgus
Angle bt. First & Second Mets.	Average	13.32	10.27
	Mean	26.00	10.50
Angle of Hallux Valgus	Average	23.37	6.45
	Mean	20.00	6.00
Angle of Met. Adductus	Average	16.08	14.27
	Mean	20.00	15.00
Angle bt. Met-Lesser Tarsus Perp.	Average	25.52	23.45
	Mean	27.00	22.50

Results

Having concluded that no axial rotation could be demonstrated in this study, the data was then correlated in search of other relationships. Table 1 lists the averages and the means taken from the dorsal-plantar radiographs. In considering the patients exhibiting hallux valgus (Figs. 12, 13) as opposed to those that do not, it must be borne in mind that there was a great disparity of ages. The average age of the group exhibiting the deformity was 59.0 while the average age of the younger group was 25.0. Despite this great difference, there was nevertheless a number of significant findings. It was clear that the angle of metatarsus adductus and the angle between the first metatarsal and the lesser tarsus perpendicular seem to show no relationship to the hallux valgus deformity. However, it was evident that the angle between the first and second metatarsals as well as the angle of hallux valgus do show a relation to the deformity and more specifically to the deviation of the sesamoids.

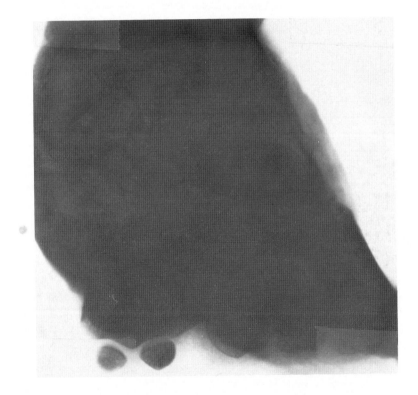

Figure 8. Patient M.P. – Normal sesamoid position.

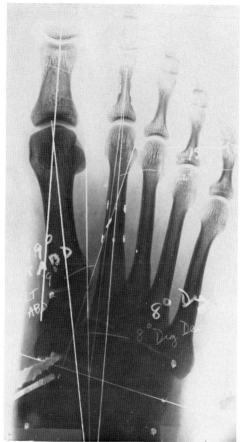

Figure 9. Patient M.P. — Normal dorsal-plantar x-ray.

The graph in Figure 14 of the angle between the first metatarsal and the proximal phalanx to the sesamoid deviation shows a more direct relation than does the graph in Figure 15 of the sesamoid deviation to the angle between the first and second metatarsals. These two angles also vary directly with each other as shown in the graph in Figure 16.

Conclusions

Using a new positioning device as described by Downey and Dorothy in their article in the April, 1969 issue of *the Journal of the American Podiatry Association*, it was shown to be possible to produce a radiographic film

Figure 10. Patient L.B. – Third degree sesamoid deviation.

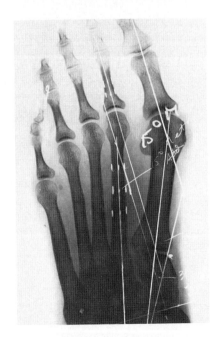

Figure 11. Patient L.B. – Moderate hallux valgus deformity.

Figure 12. Patient M.M. – Fourth degree sesamoid deviation.

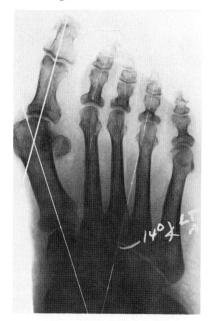

Figure 13. Patient M.M. – Severe hallux valgus deformity.

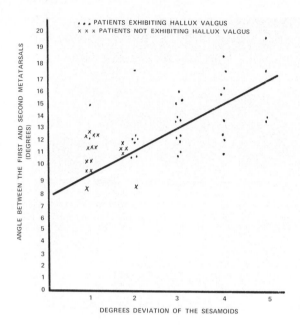

Figure 15.

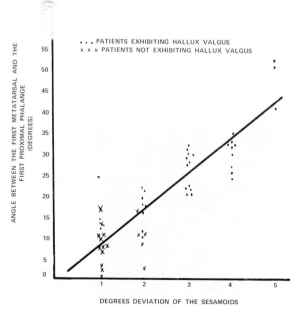

Figure 14.

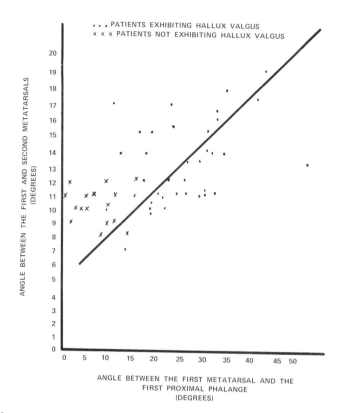

Figure 16.

demonstrating the relationship of the plantar metatarsal heads to the transverse plane. With the use of this device, it was proposed to determine the amount of axial rotation of the first metatarsal in patients with varying degrees of hallux valgus and to relate this to measurements taken from the dorsal-plantar x-rays. The survey group consisted of forty-seven cases with objectively visible hallux valgus and eleven cases with no apparent signs of the deformity.

In correlating the data, four distinct observations could be made. These are:

1. Axial rotation of the first metatarsal was not found to be significant nor measureable in this study.

2. The angle of metatarsus adductus and the angle between the first metatarsal and the lesser tarsus perpendicular showed no statistical relation to the degree of displacement of the sesamoids.

3. The angle between the first and second metatarsals and the angle of hallux valgus vary directly with each other.

4. Both the angle between the first and the second metatarsal as well as the angle of hallux valgus show a direct statistical relationship to the degree of sesamoid displacement and thus to the severity of the hallux valgus deformity.

In addition to the above-noted observations, it was also consistently noted that where there was found to be a high degree of sesamoid displacement, there was also seen an erosion of the intersesamoid ridge. Therefore, when evaluating treatment of the hallux valgus deformity, it becomes imperative that in addition to considering the angles shown in Figures 14-16 the displacement of the sesamoids must be examined with attention given to the condition of the intersesamoid ridge.

References

1. Downey, D.: A Radiographic Technique to Demonstrate the Plantar Aspect of the Forefoot in Stance, *Journal of the American Podiatry Association 59*, January 1969, pp. 140-143.
2. DuVries, H. L.: *Surgery of the Foot*. St. Louis: C. V. Mosby Company, 1959.
3. Goff, C.: Weight-Bearing X-rays of the Feet, *American Journal of Orthopedic Surgery* January, 1968, pp. 13-16.
4. Haines, M.: Anatomy of Hallux Valgus. *Journal of Bone and Joint Surgery 36B*, 1954, pp. 274-293.
5. Hall, M.: *The Locomotor System Functional Anatomy*. Illinois: Charles Thomas Company, 1965.
6. Hardy, C.: Observations on Hallux Valgus. *Journal of Bone and Joint Surgery 33B*, 1951, pp. 376-391.
7. Hardy, V.: Sources of Error in the Production and Measurement of Standing Radiographs of the Foot.*British Journal of Radiology 24*, 1951.
8. Kelikian, H.: *Hallux Valgus, Allied Deformities of the Forefoot and Metatarsalgia*. Philadelphia: W. B. Saunders Company, 1965.
9. Piggot, H.: The Natural History of Hallux Valgus in Adolescents and Early Adult Life. *Journal of Bone and Joint Surgery 42B*, 1960, pp. 740-760.
10. Sklier, J. D.: *Functional Orthopedics*. Troy, New York: 1969.

Author's Index

Addante, J. B. , 207

Collett, R. W. , 3 ·

Davis, J. A., 239
Doller, J., 143
Duhon, S. C., 109

Feldman, M. H., 185
Fulp, M., 143

Hara, B., 22
Hawkins, L. G., 15
Helms, D. C., 59
Hunt, J. H., 51
Hussar, D. A., 85

Jones, C. L., 251

Kaplan, E. G., 207
Kurowsky, J. L. 45

Levine, S., 291
Lowe, W., 22

Maldin, R. A., 305
McGlone, J. J., 199
Michota, F. A., 295
Michota, S. V., 295
Miles, J. S., 135
Moeller, F. A. . 121
Moskow, S., 97

Root, M. L., 11
Rothbart, B. A., 271

Schuster, R. P., 7
Sgarlato, T. E., 153
Shreve, C., 207
Smith, S. D., 63
Sokoloff, T. H., 129
Starks, C. R., 143

Turchin, C. R., 221

Weil, L. S., 75
Weinstock, R. E., 171

Zerr, E., 39